POINTS OF CHINESE ACUPUNCTURE

by

Dr. J. LAVIER

Physician Member, The Taipai Acupuncture Hospital,
Licentiate and Titulary Member, The College of Acupuncture,
Taipai, Formosa, Free China.
Honorary Counsellor, The Conference of Master Acupuncteurs
of the Far East.

English Edition Translated,
Indexed and Adapted
by

Dr. Philip M. Chancellor

Physician Member, The Taipai Acupuncture Hospital.
Licentiate and Titulary Member, The College of Acupuncture,
Taipai, Formosa, Free China.
Member of the Chinese Acupuncture Society, Taiwan, Formosa,
Free China.

HEALTH SCIENCE PRESS
RUSTINGTON, SUSSEX, ENGLAND

Dr. Lavier has written:

Ce Qu'il Faut Savoir sur l'Acupuncture, Paris, 1961.

and has translated from the Chinese:
Formulaire d'Acupuncture, Paris, 1959.
Théorie et Pratique de l'Acupuncture, Paris, 1960.

Dr. Chancellor has written:

The English Adaptation of Chinese Acupuncture, London, 1962.

The Song of Magic—The Sacred Runes of The Edda—An Interpretation, México, 1964.

To my parents, in respectful dedication

J. Lavier.

[illegible]

[illegible]

TABLE OF CONTENTS

PART I

PART II

PART III

PART IV

GENERAL TOPOGRAPHY OF THE MERIDIANS

The meridians and their abbreviations:

LU : meridian of the lungs, Fei Ching.
CO : meridian of the large intestine, Ch'ang Ching.
ST : meridian of the stomach, Wei Ching.
SP : meridian of the spleen,. P'i Ching.
HT : meridian of the heart, Hsin Ching.
SI : meridian of the small intestine, Hsiao Ch'ang Ching.
BL : meridian of the bladder, P'ang Kuang Ching.
KI : meridian of the kidneys, Shen Ching.
HC : meridian of the heart constrictor, Hsin, Pao Lê Ching.
TH : meridian of the tri-heaters, San Chao Ching.
GB : meridian of the gallbladder, Tan Ching.
LI : meridian of the liver,Kan Ching.
VG : meridian of the governing vessel, Tu Mei.
VC : meridian of the vessel of conception, Jen Mei.

Other abbreviations:
C : Cervical vertebra.
T : Thoracic vertebra.

Some of the diagrams have special letter-symbols to show co-ordinate points. These abbreviations are explained in the text on the page facing the drawing.

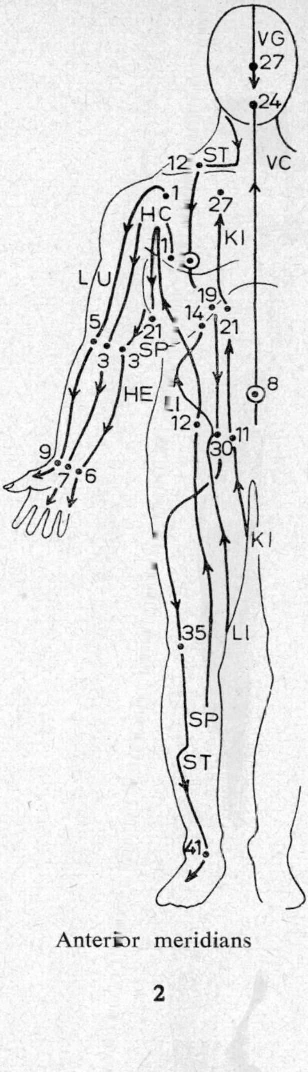

Anterior meridians

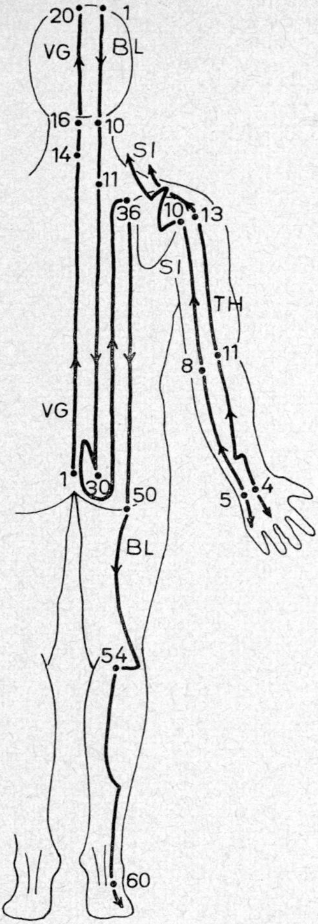

Posterior meridians

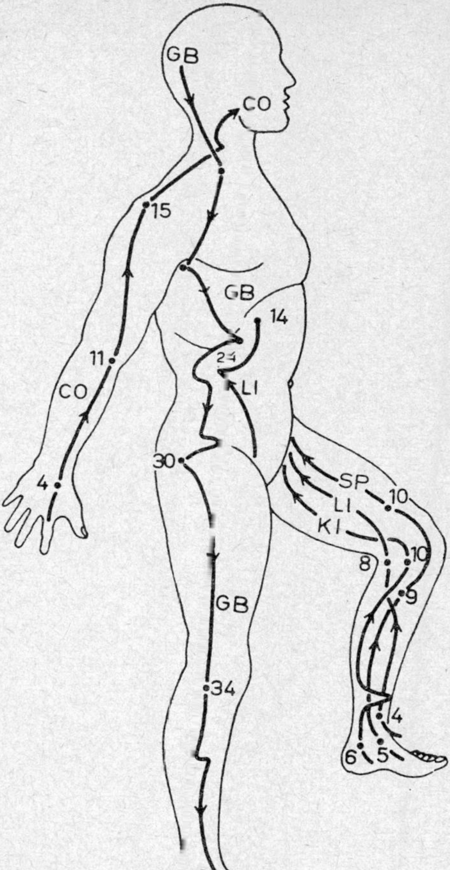

Lateral meridians

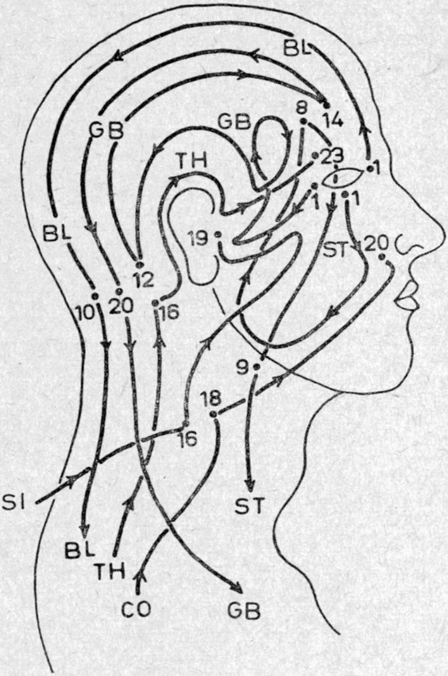

Cranial meridians

B

REGIONAL TOPOGRAPHY OF THE POINTS OF ACUPUNCTURE

The following symbols are used in the diagrams:

● Normal point for piqure or cauterizations.

■ Piqure FORBIDDEN.

△ Cauterizations FORBIDDEN.

× Piqure and cauterizations FORBIDDEN.

The maximum depth to which a piqure should be made and the maximum number of attenuated cauterizations that should be given are listed after the name of the point. These are safe limits for an adult of average weight and stature, and they should not be exceeded at any time.

ARM

ANTERIOR SURFACE

The local value for the pouce is: 1/7th part of the distance between the elbow (EL) and the "V" of the deltoideous muscle (DE).

3—LU, T'ien Fu. Piqure: 8—10 mm.
Cauterizations: FORBIDDEN.
4—LU, Hsieh Pai. Piqure: 6—10mm.
Cauterizations: 5.
5—LU, Ch'ih Chih. Piqure: 6—10 mm.
Cauterizations: 3—5.

2—HE, Ch'iang Ling. Piqure: FORBIDDEN.
Cauterizations: 5.
3—HE, Shao Hai. Piqure: 4—6 mm.
Cauterizations: 3—5.

2—HC, T'ien Ch'üan. Piqure: 10 mm.
Cauterizations: 3.
3—HC, Ch'ü Chih. Piqure: 6 mm.
Cauterizations: 5.

Note Point 1—HE is located in the armpit and is not shown on the diagram. Its characteristics are: Piqure: 10 mm. Cauterization: 5.

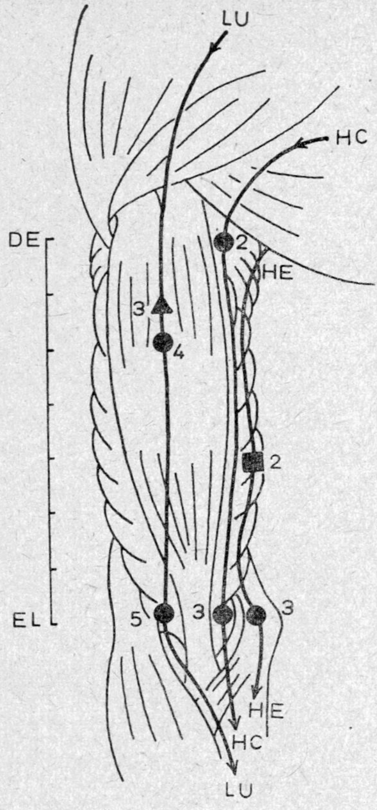

ARM, anterior surface

ARM

POSTERIOR SURFACE

The local value for the pouce is: 1/7th part of the distance between the elbow (EL) and the "V" of the deltoideus muscle (DE).

9—SI, Chien Chen. Piqure; 10—14mm.
Cauterizations: FORBIDDEN.

10—TH, T'ien Ching. Piqure: 6—10mm.
Cauterziations: 3—5.

11—TH, Ch'ing Lêng Yüan. Piqure: 6mm.
Cauterizations: 3—7.

12—TH, Hsiao Lê. Piqure: 10mm.
Cauterizations: 3—7.

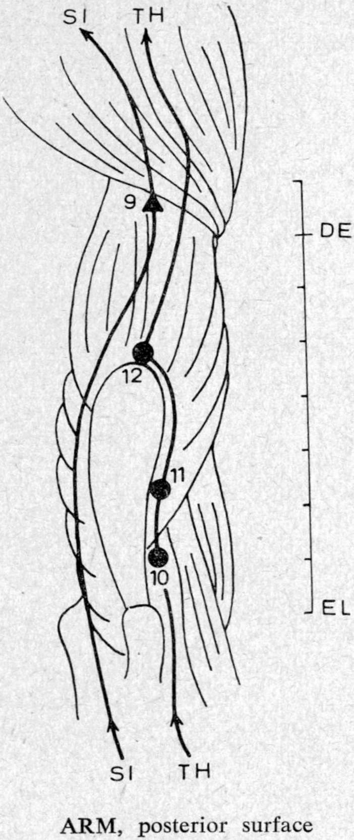

ARM, posterior surface

The local value for the pouce is: 1/7th part of the distance between the elbow (EL) and the "V" of the deltoideus muscle (DE).

11—CO, Ch'ü Ch'ih. Piqure: 10—16mm.
Cauterizations: 5—10.

12—CO, Chou Liao. Piqure: 6mm.
Cauterizations: 3.

13—CO, (Yang) Wu Li. Piqure: FORBIDDEN.
Cauterizations: 7.

14—CO, Pi Nao. Piqure: 6mm.
Cauterizations: 3—7.

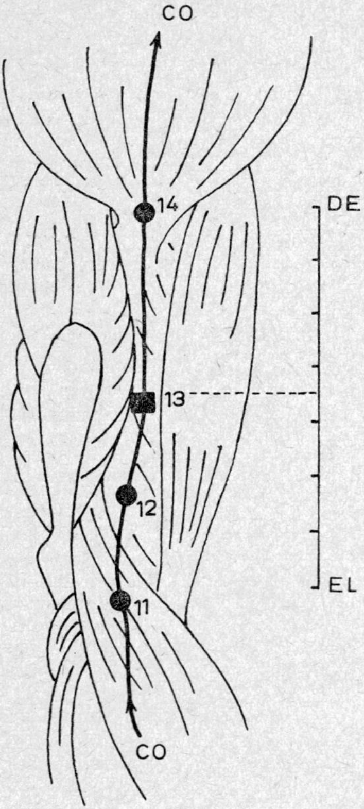

ARM, exterior surface

FOREARM

ANTERIOR SURFACE

The local value for the pouce is: 1/12th part of the distance between the elbow (EL) and the wrist (WR).

6—LU, K'ung Tsui. Piqure: 10mm.
Cauterizations: 5.
7—LU, Lieh Ch'üeh. Piqure: 4—6mm.
Cauterizations: 3—5.
8—LU, Ching Chü. Piqure: 4—6mm.
Cauterizations: FORBIDDEN.
9—LU, T'ai Yüan. Piqure: 4mm.
Cauterizations: 3.

4—HE, Ling Tao. Piqure: 6mm.
Cauterizations: 3—5.
5—HE, T'ung Li. Piqure: 6mm.
Cauterizations: 3—5.
6—HE, Yin Chi. Piqure: 6mm.
7—HE, Shen Men. Piqure: 6mm.
Cauterizations: 5—7.

4—HC, Ch'i Men. Piqure: 8mm.
Cauterizations: 5.
5—HC, Chien Shih. Piqure: 6mm.
Cauterizations: 5.
6—HC, Nei Kuan. Piqure: 6mm.
Cauterizations: 5.
7—HC, Ta Ling. Piqure: 6mm.
Cauterizations: 5—7.

Note: For points 5—LU, 3—HE and 3—HC, see ARM, anterior surface.

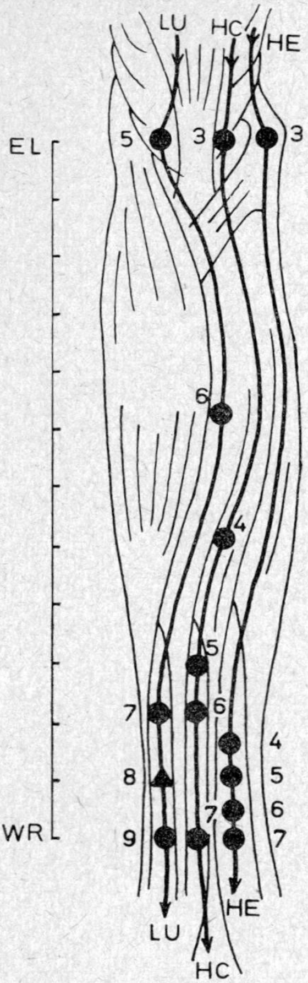

FOREARM, anterior surface

FOREARM

POSTERIOR SURFACE

The local value for the pouce is: 1/12th part of the distance between the elbow (EL) and the wrist (WR).

5—SI, Yang Ku.
Piqure: 4mm. Cauterizations: 3—5.
6—SI, Yang Lao.
Piqure: 6mm. Cauterizations: 3—5.
7—SI, Chih Cheng.
Piqure: 6mm. Cauterizations: 3—7.
8—SI, Hsiao Hai.
Piqure: 4mm. Cauterizations: 5.

4—TH, Yang Ch'ih.
Piqure: 6mm. Cauterizations: FORBIDDEN.
5—TH, Wai Luan.
Piqure: 10mm. Cauterizations: 3—7.
6—TH, Chih Kou.
Piqure: 10mm. Cauterizations: 5.
7—TH, Hui Tsung.
Piqure: 6mm. Cauterizations: 5—7.
8—TH, San Yang Lê.
Piqure: FORBIDDEN. Cauterizations: 7.
9—TH, Ssŭ Tu.
Piqure: 12mm. Cauterizations: 3—7.

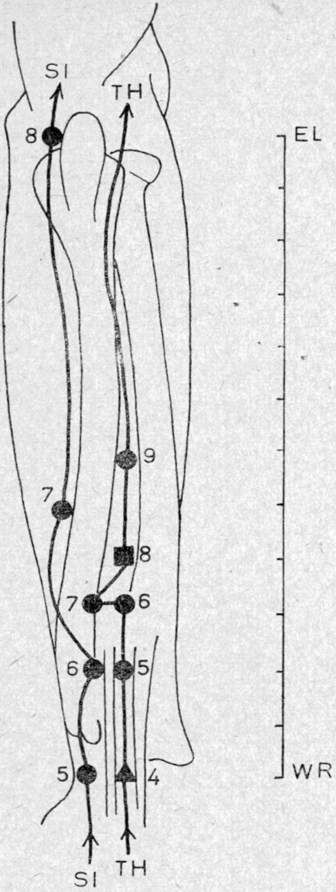

FOREARM, posterior surface

FOREARM

EXTERIOR SURFACE

The local value for the pouce is: 1/12th part of the distance between the elbow (EL) and the wrist (WR).

5—CO, Yang Ch'i.
Piqure: 6mm. Cauterizations: 5.
6—CO, Pi'en Li.
Piqure: 6mm. Cauterizations: 5—7.
7—CO, Wen Liu.
Piqure: 6mm. Cauterizations: 5—30.
8—CO, (Shou) Hsia Lien.
Piqure: 8mm. Cauterizations: 6.
9—CO, (Shou) Shang Lien.
Piqure: 8mm. Cauterizations: 5—10.
10—CO, (Shou) San Li.
Piqure: 10mm. Cauterizations: 5—10.
11—CO, Ch'ü Ch'ih.
Piqure: 10—16mm. Cauterizations: 5—10.

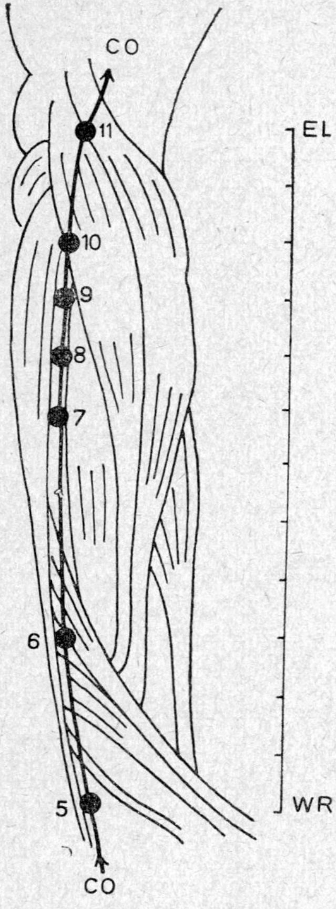

FOREARM, exterior surface

PALMAR SURFACE

10—LU, Yü Chi.
Piqure: 6—10mm. Cauterizations: FORBIDDEN.

8—HE, Shao Fu.
Piqure: 6mm. Cauterizations: 3—5.

8—HC, Lao Kung.
Piqure: 4—6mm. Cauterizations: 3.

Note: For points 9—LU, 7—HE and 7—HC, see FOREARM, anterior surface.

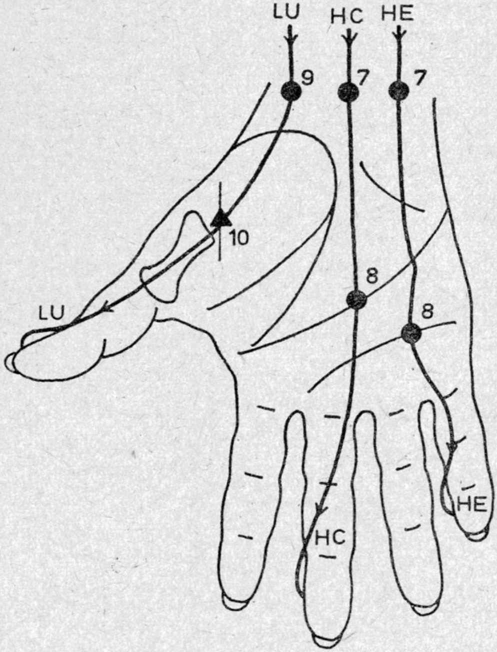

HAND, palmar surface

HAND
DORSAL SURFACE

1—CO, Shang Yang.
Piqure: 2mm. Cauterizations: 3.

2—CO, Erh Chien.
Piqure: 6mm. Cauterizations: 3.

3—CO, San Chien.
Piqure: 6mm. Cauterizations: 3.

4—CO, Ho Ku.
Piqure: 10mm. Cauterizations: 5—7.

1—SI, Shao Chih.
Piqure: 2mm. Cauterizations: 3—5.

2—SI, Ch'ien Ku.
Piqure: 2mm. Cauterizations: 3.

3—SI, Hou Ch'i.
Piqure: 6mm. Cauterizatoins: 3—5.

4—SI, Wan Ku.
Piqure: 6mm. Cauterizations: 3—7.

1—TH, Kuan Chung.
Piqure: 2mm. Cauterizations: 3.

2—TH, Yeh Men.
Piqure: 2mm. Cauterizations: 3.

3—TH, Chang Chu.
Piqure: 6mm. Cauterizations: 3—5.

11—LU, Shao Shang.
Piqure: 2mm. Cauterizations: FORBIDDEN.

9—HE, Shao Ch'ung.
Piqure: 2mm. Cauterizations: 3—5.

9—HC, Chung Heng.
Piqure: 2mm. Cauterizations: 3.

Note: For points 5—SI and 4—TH, see FOREARM, posterior surface. For point 5—CO, see FOREARM, external surface.

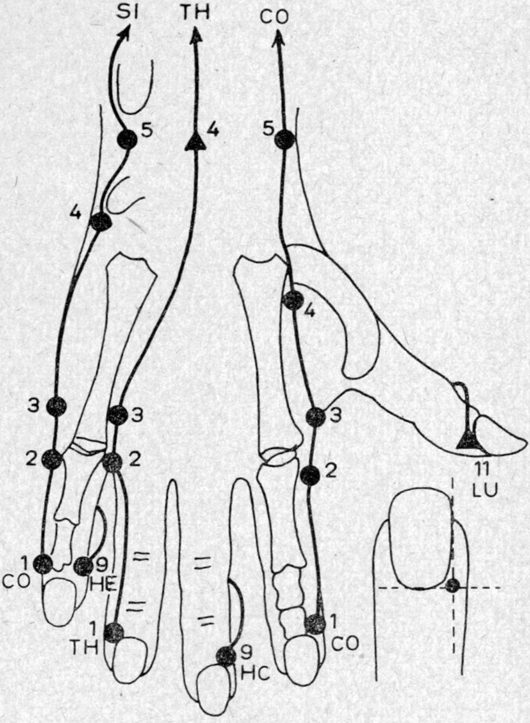

HAND, dorsal surface

THIGH

ANTERIOR SURFACE

The local value for the pouce is: 1/13th part of the distance between the great trochanter (TR) and the posterior crease of the knee (KN).

31—ST, Pi Kuan.
Piqure: 12 mm. Cauterizations: 3—7.
32—ST, Fu Tu.
Piqure: 12mm. Cauterizations: 3—7.
33—ST, Yin Shih.
Piqure: 8mm. Cauterizations: 3—5.
34—ST, Liang Ch'iu.
Piqure: 8mm. Cauterizations: 3—5.
35—ST, Tu Pi.
Piqure: 6mm. Cauterizations: 3.

11—SP, Chi Men.
Piqure: 10mm. Cauterizations: 3.

10—LI, (Yin) Wu Li.
Piqure: 10mm. Cauterizations: 5.

Note: For points 11—LI, 12—LI and 12—SP, see ABDOMEN. For point 10—SP, see THIGH, internal surface.

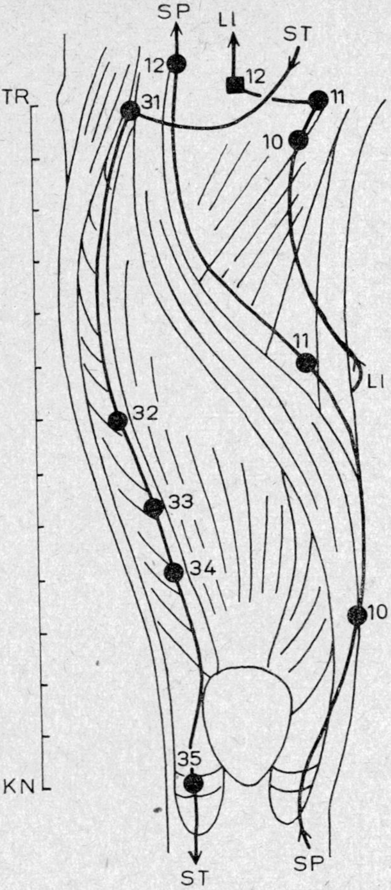

THIGH, anterior surface

THIGH

POSTERIOR SURFACE

The local value for the pouce is: 1/13th part of the distance beteween the great trochantar (TR) and the posterior crease of the knee (KN).

50—BL, Ch'eng Fu.
Piqure: 16mm. Cauterizations: FORBIDDEN.
51—BL, Yin Men.
Piqure: 14mm. Cauterizations: FORBIDDEN.
52—BL, Fou Ch'i.
Piqure: 10mm. Cauterizations: 3—7.
53—BL, Wei Yang.
Piqure: 14mm. Cauterizations: 3—5.
54—BL, Wei Chung.
Piqure: 10mm. Cauterizations: FORBIDDEN.

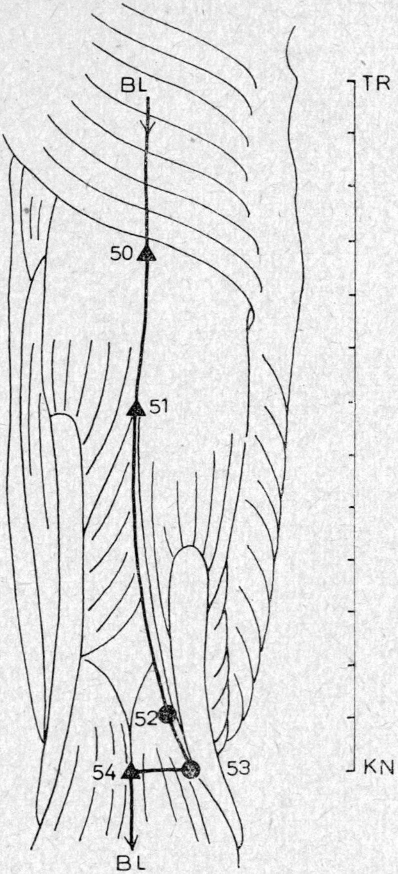

THIGH, posterior surface

THIGH

EXTERIOR SURFACE

The local value for the pouce is: 1/13th part of the distance between the grand trochantar (TR) and the posterior crease of the knee (KN).

30—GB, Huan T'iao.
Piqure: 20—30mm. Cauterizations: 7—20.
31—GB, Fêng Shih.
Piqure: 10mm. Cauterizations: 5.
32—GB, Chung Tu.
Piqure: 10mm. Cauterizations: 5—7.
33—GB, Yang Kuan.
Piqure: 10mm. Cauterizations: FORBIDDEN.

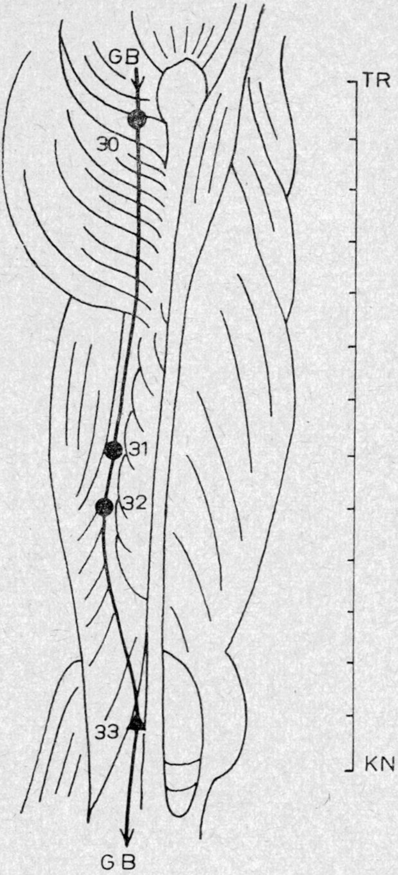

THIGH, exterior surface

THIGH

INTERIOR SURFACE

The local value for the pouce is: 1/13th part of the distance between the great trochantar (TR) and the posterior crease of the knee (KN).

10—SP, Hsüeh Hai.
Piqure: 6—10 mm. Cauterizations: 3—7.

10—KI, Yin Ku.
Piqure: 8mm. Cauterizations: 3.

8—LI, Ch'ü Ch'üan.
Piqure: 12mm. Cauterizations: 3—5.

9—LI, Yin Pao.
Piqure: 10mm. Cauterizations: 3.

Note: For point 11--SP, see THIGH, anterior surface.

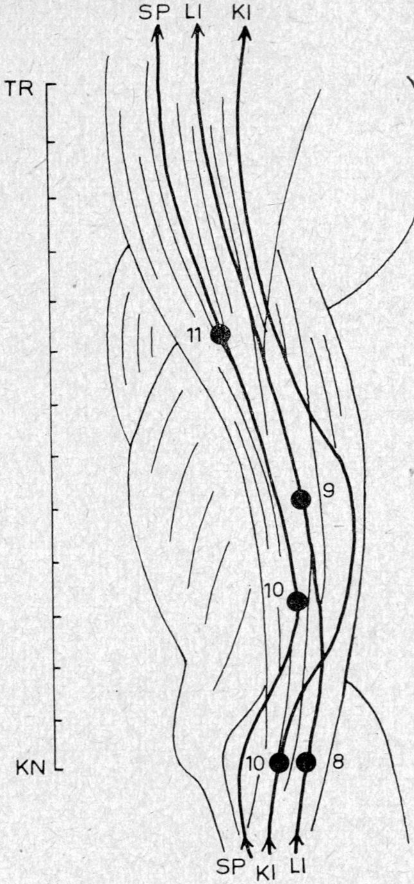

THIGH, interior surface

LEG

ANTERIOR SURFACE

The local value for the pouce is: 1/15th part of the distance between the posterior crease of the knee (KN) and the point of the interior malleolus (IM). The point of the exterior malleolus (EM) is one pouce below the point (IM).

36—ST, (Tsu) San Li.
Piqure: 10—16mm. Cauterizations: 7—20.
Cauterizations: FORBIDDEN for children less than seven years old.

37—ST,(Tsu) Shang Lien.
Piqure: 10mm. Cauterizations: 3—7.
38—ST, T'iao K'ou.
Piqure: 10mm. Cauterizations: 3—7.
39—ST, (Tsu) Hsia Lien.
Piqure: 10mm. Cauterizations: 3—7.
40—ST, Fêng Lung.
Piqure: 6mm. Cauterizations: 3—5.
41—ST, Chieh Ch'i.
Piqure: 10mm. Cauterizations: 3—7.

Note: For point 35—ST, see THIGH, anterior surface.

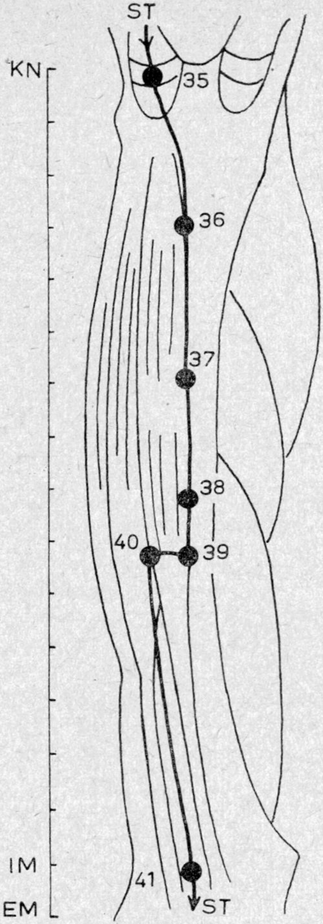

LEG, anterior surface

LEG

POSTERIOR SURFACE

The local value for the pouce is: 1/15th part of the distance between the posterior crease of the knee (KN) and the point of the interior malleolus (IM). The point of the exterior malleolus (BM) is one pouce below the point (IM).

55—BL, Ho Yang.
Piqure: 10mm. Cauterizations: 5—7.
56—BL, Ch'eng Chin.
Piqure: FORBIDDEN. Cauterizations: 3—7.
75—BL, Ch'eng Shan.
Piqure: 14mm. Cauterizations: 5—15.

Note: For points 53—BL and 54—BL, see THIGH, posterior surface. For point 58—BL, see LEG, exterior surface.

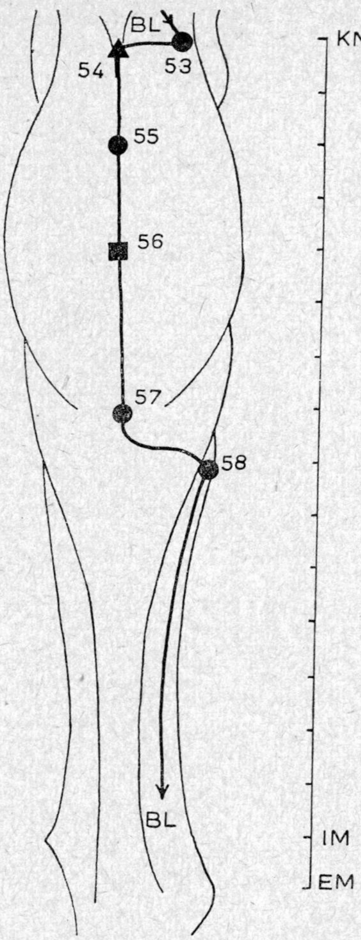

LEG, posterior surface

LEGS

EXTERIOR SURFACE

The local value for the pouce is: 1/15th part of the distance between the posterior crease of the knee (KN) and the point of the interior malleolus (IM). The point of the exterior malleolus (EM) is one pouce below the point (IM).

34—GB, Yang Ling Ch'üan.
Piqure: 12mm. Cauterizations: 7—10.
35—GB, Yang Chiao.
Piqure: 12mm. Cauterizations: 3—7.
36—GB, Wai Ch'iu.
Piqure: 8mm. Cauterizations: 3.
37—GB, Kuang Ming.
Piqure: 12mm. Cauterizations: 7.
38—GB, Yang Fu.
Piqure: 12mm. Cauterizations: 5—15.
39—GB, Hsüan Chung.
Piqure: 12mm. Cauterizations: 5—15.

58—BL, Fei Yang.
Piqure: 10mm. Cauterizations: 3—7.
59—BL, Fu Yang.
Piqure: 10mm. Cauterizations: 5—7.

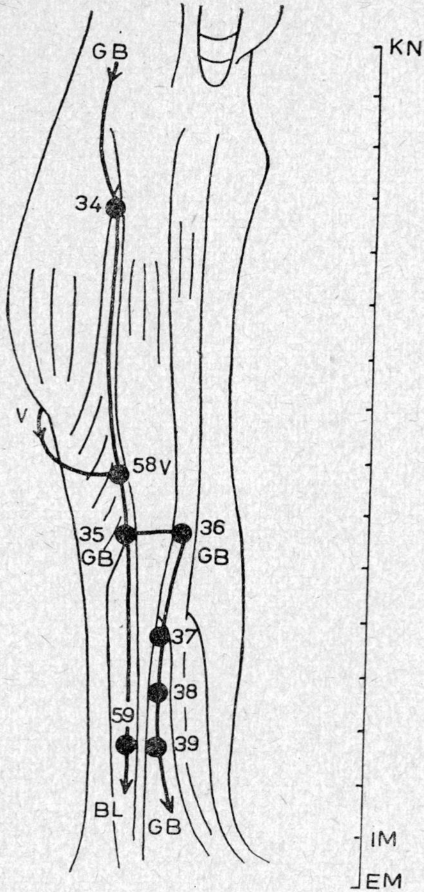

LEG, exterior surface

D

LEG

INTERIOR SURFACE

The local value for the pouce is: 1/15th part of the distance between the crease of the knee (KN) and the tip of the interior malleolus (IM). The tip of the exterior malleolus (EM) is one pouce below the point (IM).

6—SP, San Yin Chao.
Piqure: 8mm. Cauterizations: 3—10.
7—SP, Lou Ku.
Piqure: 8mm. Cauterizations: FORBIDDEN.
8—SP, Ti Chi.
Piqure: 8mm. Cauterizations: 3—7.
9—SP, Yin Ling Ch'üan.
Piqure: 10—16mm. Cauterizations: FORBIDDEN.

7—KI, Fu Liu.
Piqure: 8mm. Cauterizations: 3—7.
8—KI, Chiao Hsin.
Piqure: 6mm. Cauterizations: 5.
9—KI, Chu Pin.
Piqure: 10mm. Cauterizations: 3—7.

5—LI, Li Kou.
Piqure: 6mm. Cauterizations: 3—7.
6—LI, Chung Tu.
Piqure: 6mm. Cauterizations: 3.
7—LI, Hsi Kuan.
Piqure: 8mm. Cauterizations: 5.

Note: For points 10—KI and 8—LI, see THIGH, interior surface.

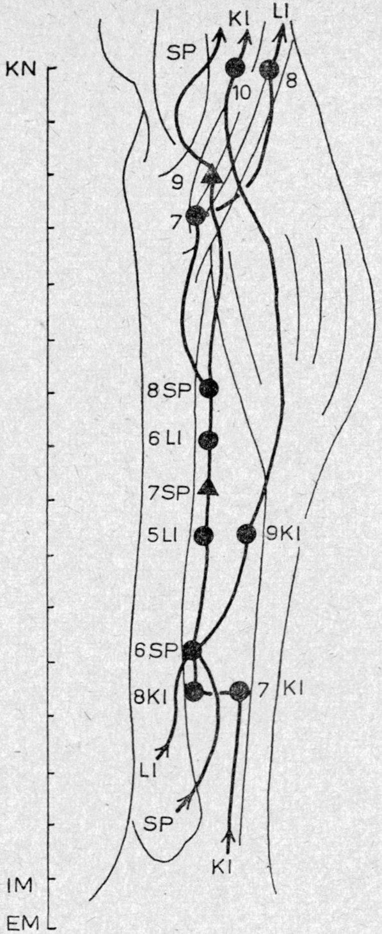

LEG, interior surface

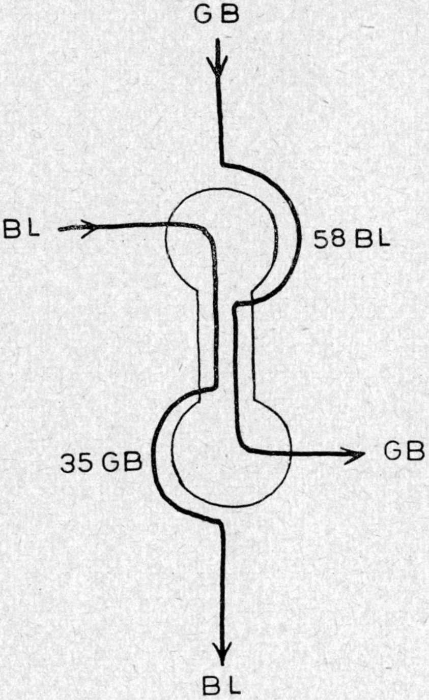

Cross-point of the Yang meridians on the exterior surface of the LEG

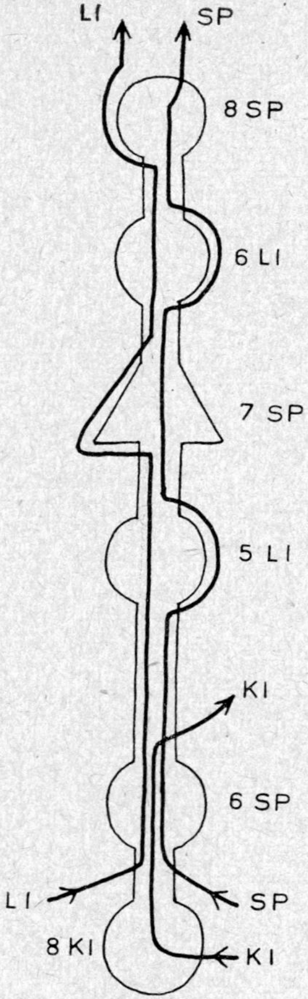

Cross-point of the Yin meridians on the interior surface of the LEG

FOOT

DORSAL SURFACE

42—ST. Ch'ung Yang.
Piqure: 6mm. Cauterizations: 3—5.
43—ST, Hsieu Ku.
Piqure: 6mm. Cauterizations: 3.
44—ST, Nei T'ing.
Piqure: 6mm. Cauterizations: 5.
45—ST, Li Tui.
Piqure: 2mm. Cauterizations: 3.

41—GB, (Tsu) Lin Ch'i.
Piqure: 5mm. Cauterizations: 5.
42—GB, Ti Wu Hui.
Piqure: 4mm. Cauterizations: FORBIDDEN.
43—GB, Hsieh Ch'i.
Piqure: 6mm. Cauterizations: 3—5.
44—GB, (Tsu) Ch'iao Yin.
Piqure: 2mm. Cauterizations: 3—5.

1—LI, Ta Tun.
Piqure: 2mm. Cauterizations: 5—7.
2—LI, Hsing Chien.
Piqure: 6mm. Cauterizations: 5—7.
3—LI, T'ai Ch'ung.
Piqure: 6mm. Cauterizations: 3—7.
4—LI, Chung Fêng.
Piqure: 8mm. Cauterizations: 3—5.

Note: For point 41—ST, see LEG, anterior surface. For point 67—BL, see FOOT, exterior surface. For point 1—SP, see FOOT, interior surface.

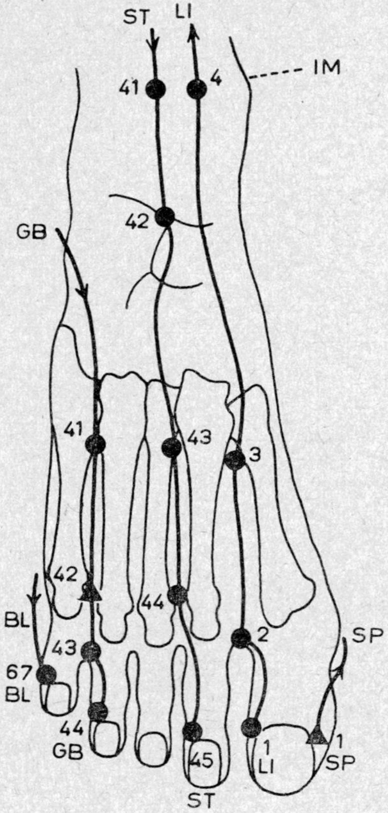

FOOT, dorsal surface

FOOT

EXTERIOR SURFACE

60—BL, Kun Lun.
Piqure: 6—10 mm. Cauterizations: 3—7.
61—BL, Pu Ts'an.
Piqure: 6mm. Cauterizations: 3—7.
62—BL, Shen Mei.
Piqure: 6mm. Cauterizations: FORBIDDEN.
63—BL, Chin Men.
Piqure: 6mm. Cauterizations: 3—5.
64—BL, Ching Ku.
Piqure: 6—10mm. Cauterizations: 3—7.
65—BL, Shu Ku.
Piqure: 6mm. Cauterizations: 3—5.
66—BL, (Yang) T'ung Ku.
Piqure: 4mm. Cauterizations: 3—5.
67—BL, Chih Yin.
Piqure: 4mm. Cauterizations: 3.

40—GB, Ch'iu Ch'ü.
Piqure: 10mm. Cauterizations: 3—7.

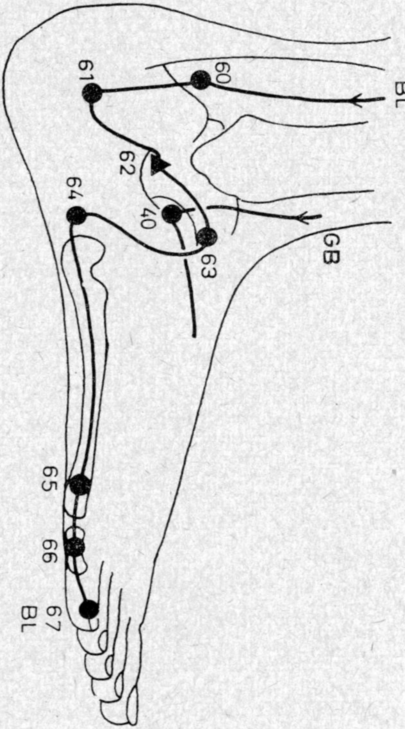

FOOT, exterior surface

FOOT

INTERIOR SURFACE

1—SP, Yin Pi.
Piqure: 2mm. Note: Piqure is absolutely FORBIDDEN in the case of pregnancy.
Cauterizations: FORBIDDEN.

2—SP (Tsu) Ta Tu.
Piqure: 6mm. Cauterizations: 3—5.
Note: Cauterization is absolutely FORBIDDEN in the case of pregnancy.

3—SP, T'ai Pai.
Piqure: 6mm. Cauterizations:3—5.

4—SP, Kung Sun.
Piqure: 6mm. Cauterizations: 3.

5—SP, Shang Ch'iu.
Piqure: 6mm. Cauterizations: 3—7.

2—KI, Jan Ku.
Piqure: 10mm. Cauterizations: 3—5.

3—KI, T'ai Ch'i.
Piqure: 6mm. Cauterizations: 3—5.

4—KI, Ta Chung.
Piqure: 6mm. Cauterizations: 3—7.

5—KI, Shui Ch'üan.
Piqure: 8mm. Cauterizations: 5.

6—KI, Chao Hai.
Piqure: 6mm. Cauterizations: 3—5.

Note: Point 1—KI is located on the sole of the foot and is not shown on the diagram. Its characteristics are:
Piqure: 10mm. Do not allow to bleed.
Cauterizations: 3—7.

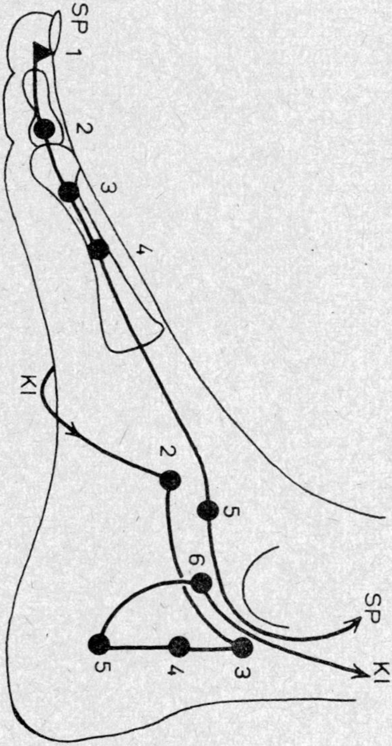

FOOT, interior surface

THORAX

The meridian of the vessel of conception (VC) lies on the median line of the thorax. The meridian of the stomach (ST) lies in line with the nipple on the thorax and is bi-lateral. The meridian of the kidneys (KI) lies between the lines of VC and ST and is bi-lateral. The points KI, ST, and SP are in the intercostal spaces; those of VC are on the sternum, on a prolongation of the line formed by the other points.

16—VC, Chung T'ing. Piqure: 6mm. Cauterizations: 5.
17—VC, Hsien Chung.
Piqure: FORBIDDEN. Cauterizations: 2.
18—VC, Yü T'ang. Piqure: 6mm. Cauterizations: 5.
19—VC, Tzü Kung. Piqure: 6mm. Cauterizations: 5.
20—VC, Hua Kai. Piqure: 6mm. Cauterizations: 6.

22—KI, Pu Lang. Piqure: 6mm. Cauterizations: 5.
23—KI, Shen Fêng. Piqure: 6mm. Cauterizations: 5.
24—KI, Ling Chü. Piqure: 6mm. Cauterizations: 5.
25—KI, Shen Ts'ang. Piqure: 6mm. Cauterizations: 5.
26—KI, Huo Chung. Piqure: 6mm. Cauterizations: 5.
27—KI, Yü Fu. Piqure: 6mm. Cauterizations: 5.

13—ST, Ch'i Hu. Piqure: 6mm. Cauterizations: 5.
14—ST, K'u Fang. Piqure: 6mm. Cauterizations: 5.
15—ST, Wu I. Piqure: 6mm. Cauterizations: 5.
16—ST, Ying Ch'uang. Piqure: 6mm. Cauterizations: 5.
17—ST, Ju Chung.
Piqure: FORBIDDEN. Cauterizations: FORBIDDEN.
18—ST, Ju Ken. Piqure: 6mm. Cauterizations: 3—5.

17—SP, Shih Tou. Piqure: 6mm. Cauterizations: 5.
18—SP, T'ien Ch'i. Piqure: 6mm. Cauterizations: 5.
19—SP, Hsiung Hsiang. Piqure: 6mm. Cauterizations: 5.
20—SP, Chou Jung. Piqure: 6mm. Cauterizations: 5.

1—HC, T'ien Ch'ih. Piqure: 6mm. Cauterizations: 3—5.

Note: For point 15—VC, see EPIGASTRIUM. For point 21—VC, see NECK AND SHOULDER, anterior surface.

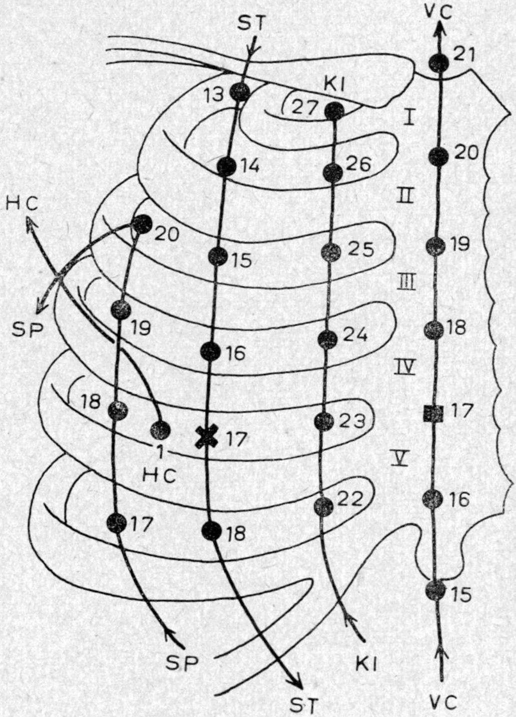

ST
VC
21
KI
13
27
I
20
14
26
II
HC
20
25
19
15
III
SP
19
24
18
16
IV
17
18
23
17
1
HC
V
22
16
17
18
15
SP
ST
KI
VC

THORAX

EPIGASTRIUM

The horizontal value for the pouce is: 1/42nd part of the circumference of the body measured at the waist. The vertical value for the pouce is: 1/7th part of the distance between the tip of the xiphoid process (XI) and the umbilicus (UM).

8—VC, Shen Ch'üeh.
Piqure: FORBIDDEN. Cauterizations: 3—30. (with salt).
9—VC, Shui Fen. Piqure: 10mm. Cauterizations 5—15.
10—VC, Hsia Kuan. Piqure: 16mm. Cauterizations: 7/15.
11—VC, Chien Li.
Piqure: 10—16mm. Cauterizations: 5—15.
12—VC, Chung Kuan.
Piqure: 6—16mm. Cauterizations: 7—15.
13—VC, Shang Kuan.
Piqure: 12mm. Cauterizations: 7—15.
14—VC, Chü Ch'üeh.
Piqure: 12mm. Cauterizations: 7—15.
15—VC, Chiu Wei.
Piqure: 6—10 mm. Cauterizations: 3—5.

16—KI, Huang Yü. Piqure. 20mm. Cauterizations: 7.
17—KI, Shang Ch'ü. Piqure: 20mm. Cauterizations: 7.
18—KI, Shih Kuan. Piqure: 14—10mm. Cauterizations: 7.
19—KI, Yin Tu.
Piqure: 14—20mm. Cauterizations: 7—10.
20—KI, Yin T'ung Ku.
Piqure: 10mm. Cauterizations: 7—10.
21—KI, Yu Men. Piqure: 10mm. Cauterizations: 7—10.

19—ST, Pu Yung. Piqure: 10mm. Cauterizations: 3—7.
20—ST, Ch'eng Men. Piqure: 10mm. Cauterizations: 3—7.
21—ST, Liang Men. Piqure: 14mm. Cauterizations: 5—15.
22—ST, Kuan Men. Piqure: 16mm. Cauterizations: 5—15.
23—ST, T'ai I. Piqure: 16mm. Cauterizations: 5—10.
24—ST, Hu Ju Men. Piqure: 16mm. Cauterizations: 5.15.
25—ST, T'ien Ch'u. Piqure: 10mm. Cauterizations: 5—20.

15—SP, Ta Hung. Piqure: 20mm. Cauterizations: 5—10.
16—SP, Fu Ai. Piqure: 14mm. Cauterizations: 5—10.

14—LI, Ch'i Men. Piqure: 8mm. Cauterizations: 5—7.

24—GB, Jih Yüeh. Piqure: 10mm. Cauterizations: 5—7.

Note: For point 13—LI, see TRUNK, lateral surface.

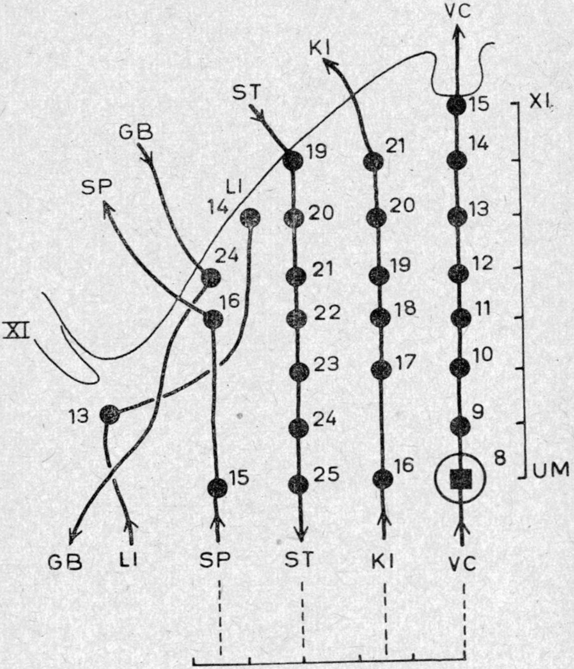

EPIGASTRIUM

ABDOMEN

The horizontal value for the pouce is: 1/42nd part of the circumference of the body measured at the waist. The vertical value for the pouce is: 1/5th part of the distance between the umbilicus (UM) and the upper edge of the pubis (PU). (GR) is the crease of the groin.

2—VC, Ch'ü Ku. Piqure: 10mm. Cauterizations: 7.
3—VC, Chuang Chi.
Piqure: 16mm. Cauterizations: 5—15.
4—VC, Kuan Yüen.
Piqure: 20—30mm. Cauterizations: 7—15.
Cauterizations forbidden prior to micturition.
5—VC, Shih Men.
Piqure: 14—16mm. Cauterizations: 7—15.
6—VC, Ch'i Hai. Piqure: 16mm. Cauterizations: 7—15.
7—VC, Yin Chiao. Piqure: 16mm. Cauterizations: 7.

11—KI, Hung Ku.
Piqure: FORBIDDEN. Cauterizations: 5—15.
12—KI, Ta Ho. Piqure: 10—20mm. Cauterizations: 5—10.
13—KI, Ch'i Hsüeh.
Piqure: 10—20mm. Cauterizations: 7—10.
14—KI, Ssu Man.
Piqure: 14—10mm. Cauterizations: 5—30.
15—KI, Chung Chu.
Piqure: 14—20mm. Cauterizations: 5—15.

26—ST, Wai Ling. Piqure 10mm. Cauterizations: 5.
27—ST, Ta Chü.
Piqure: 16—20mm. Cauterizations: 5—10.
28—ST, Shui Tao. Piqure: 16mm. Cauterizations: 5—10.
29—ST, Kuei Lai. Piqure: 10mm. Cauterizations: 5—10.
30—ST, Ch'i Ch'ung. Piqure: 6mm. Cauterizations: 7.

12—SP, Ch'ung Men. Piqure: 13mm. Cauterizations: 5.
13—SP, Fu Shê. Piqure: 14mm. Cauterizations: 5—10.
14—SP, Fu Chieh. Piqure: 14mm. Cauterizations: 5—10.

11—LI, Yin Lien. Piqure: 6mm. Cauterizations: 5.
12—LI, Ch'i Men.
Piqure: FORBIDDEN. Cauterizations: 3.

Note: For the points 15—SP, 25—ST, 16—KI and 8—VC, see EPIGASTRIUM. Point 1—VC is located upon the centre of the perineum and is not shown on the diagram. Its characteristics are: Piqure: 20mm. Cauterizations: FORBIDDEN.

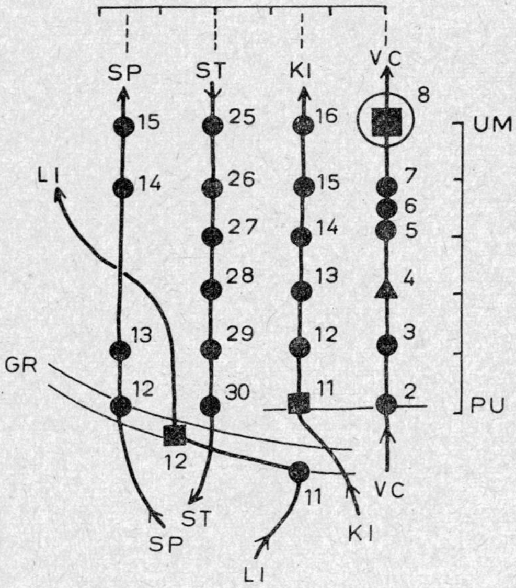
SP
ST
KI
VC
15
25
16
8
UM
LI
14
26
15
7
6
5
27
14
28
13
4
13
29
12
3
GR
12
30
11
2
PU
12
11
VC
ST
SP
KI
LI

ABDOMEN

E

TORSO

LATERAL SURFACE

The points of reference are: the line of the axilla, the inter-costal spaces, the points on the 11th and 12th ribs, and the co-ordinates shown on the diagram where (TR) is the great trochantar.

22—GB, Yüen I.
Piqure: 8mm. Cauterizations: FORBIDDEN.
23—GB, Chih Chin.
Piqure: 10mm. Cauterizations: 5.
24—GB, Jih Yüeh.
Piqure: 10mm. Cauterizations: 5—7.
25—GB, Ching Men.
Piqure: 14mm. Cauterizations: 7—12.
26—GB, Tai Mei.
Piqure: 16mm. Cauterizations: 5—15.
27—GB, Wu Ch'u.
Piqure: 14mm. Cauterizations: 3—10.
28—GB, Wei Tao.
Piqure: 16mm. Cauterizations: 5—7.
29—GB, Chü Liao.
Piqure: 16mm. Cauterizations: 5—7.

13—LI, Chang Men.
Piqure: 12—16mm. Cauterizations: 7—20.
14—LI, Ch'i Men. Piqure: 8mm. Cauterizations: 5—7.

21—SP, Ta Pao.
Piqure: 6mm. Cauterizations: 3—7.

Note: For point 24—GB, see EPIGASTRIUM. For point 30—GB, see THIGH, exterior surface.

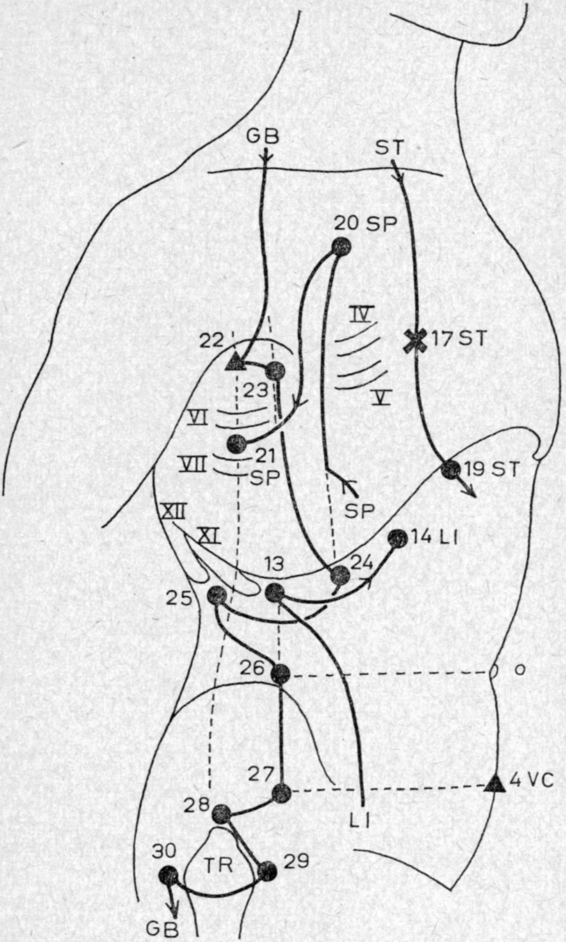

TORSO, lateral surface

TORSO

UPPER DORSAL SURFACE

The meridian of the governing vessel (VG) lies upon the median line. The meridian of the bladder (BL) is formed by two parallel vertical lines; one touches the inner edge of the scapula and the other is midway between the edge of the scapula and the median line.

9—VG, Chih Yang. Piqure: 10mm. Cauterizations:7.
10—VG, Ling T'ai.
Piqure: FORBIDDEN. Cauterizations: 3—7.
11—VG, Shen Tao.
Piqure: FORBIDDEN. Cauterizations: 3.
12—VG, Shen Chu.
Piqure: 8mm. Cauterizations: 5—30.
13—VG, T'ao Tao. ...
Piqure: 8mm. Cauterizations: 5.
14—VG, Ta Chui.
Piqure: 8mm. Cauterizations: 5—15.
11—BL, Ta Chu.
Piqure: 6mm. Cauterizations: 7.
12—BL, Fêng. Men.
Piqure: 10mm. Cauterizations: 5—10.
13—BL, Fei Yü.
Piqure: 6—10mm. Cauterizations: 7—20.
14—BL, Chüêh Yin Yü.
Piqure: 6mm. Cauterizations: 7.
15—BL, Hsin Yü.
Piqure: 6mm. Cauterizations: 3.
16—BL, Tu Chü.
Piqure: FORBIDDEN. Cauterizations: 3.
17—BL, Ko Yü.
Piqure: 8mm. Cauterizations: 7—20.
36—BL, Fu Fen.
Piqure: 8mm. Cauterizations: 7.
37—BL, P'ei Hu.
Piqure: 10mm. Cauterizations: 7—15.
38—BL, Kao Huang.
Piqure: 6mm. Cauterizations: 7—50.
39—BL, Shen T'ang.
Piqure: 6mm. Cauterizations: 5.
40—BL, I Hsi.
Piqure: 6mm. Cauterizations: 5—15.
41—BL, Ko Kuan.
Piqure: 10mm. Cauterizations: 3—15.

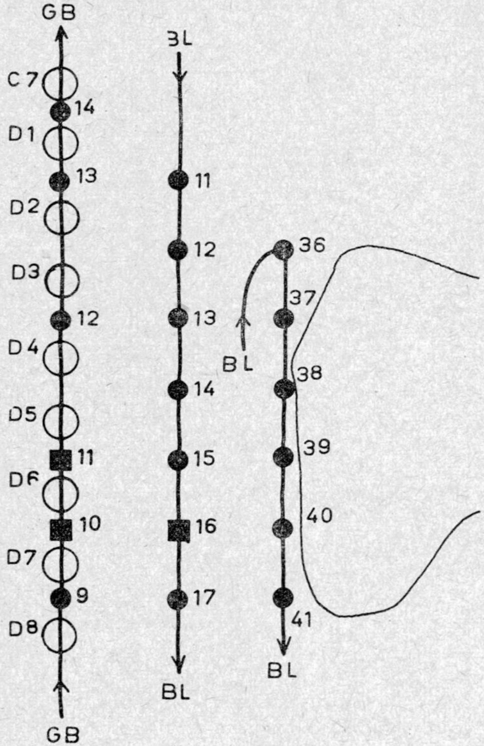

TORSO, upper dorsal surface

TORSO

DORSO-LUMBAR SURFACE

The meridian of the governing vessel (VG) lies upon the median line. The meridian of the bladder (BL) is formed by two parallel vertical lines; one touches the inner edge of the scapula and the other is midway between the edge of the scapula and the median line.

4—VG, Ming Men.
Piqure: 6mm. Cauterizations: 7—15.
5—VG, Hsüan Ch'u.
Piqure: 6mm. Cauterizations: 7—15.
6—VG, Chi Chung.
Piqure: 6mm. Cauterizations: FORBIDDEN.
7—VG, Chung Ch'u.
Piqure: FORBIDDEN.
Cauterizations: FORBIDDEN.
8—VG, Chin Shu.
Piqure: 8mm. Cauterizations: 3.
18—BL, Kan Yü.
Piqure: 3mm. Cauterizations: 7—20.
19—BL, Tan Yü.
Piqure: 6—10mm. Cauterizations: 3—15.
20—BL, P'i Yü.
Piqure: 6—10mm. Cauterizations: 7—20.
21—BL, Wei Yü.
Piqure: 6—10mm. Cauterizations: 7—21.
22—BL, San Chiao Yü.
Piqure: 6—10mm. Cauterizations: 7—20.
23—BL, Shen Yü.
Piqure: 10—16mm. Cauterizations: 3—15.
42—BL, Hun Men.
Piqure: 10mm. Cauterizations: 3—15.
43—BL, Yang Kang.
Piqure: 10mm. Cauterizations: 5.
44—BL, I She.
Piqure: 10—14mm. Cauterizations: 5—15.
45—BL, Wei Ts'ang.
Piqure: 10—14mm. Cauterizations: 5—10.
46—BL, Huang Men.
Piqure: 10—14mm. Cauterizations: 7—15.
47—BL, Chih Shih.
Piqure: 14—18mm. Cauterizations: 7—15.

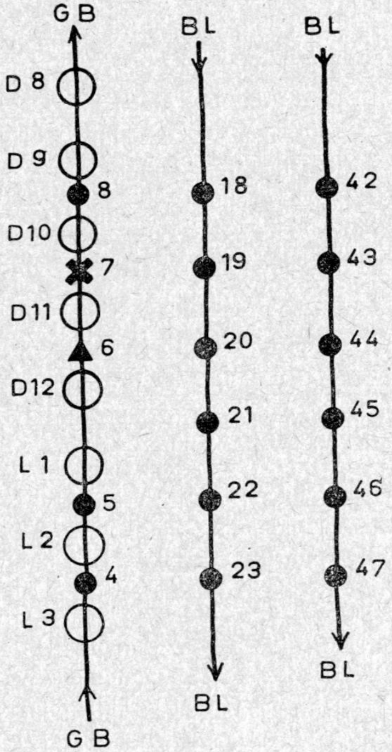

TORSO, dorsal-lumbar surface

TORSO

SACRO-LUMBAR SURFACE

The meridian of the governing vessel (VG) lies upon the median line. The meridian of the bladder (BL) is formed by two parallel vertical lines; one touches the inner edge of the scapula and the other is midway between the edge of the scapula and the median line. The middle line descends to point 30—BL, where it reverses itself to pass through the points of the sacral foramen.

1—VG, Ch'ang Ch'iang.
Piqure: 6mm. Cauterizations: 5—20.
2—VG, Yau Yü.
Piqure: 6—16mm. Cauterizations: 5—15.
3—VG, Yang Kuan.
Piqure: 6—16mm. Cauterizations: 5—15.

24—BL, Chi Hai Yü.
Piqure: 10mm. Cauterizations: 3—5.
25—BL, Ta Ch'ang Yü.
Piqure: 16—20mm. Cauterizations: 7—20.
26—BL, Kuan Yüan Yü.
Piqure: 20mm. Cauterizations: 3.
27—BL, Hsiao Ch'ang Yü.
Piqure: 16—20mm. Cauterizations: 7—20.
28—BL, P'ang Kuang Yü.
Piqure: 16—20mm. Cauterizations: 7—15.
29—BL, Chung T'un Yü.
Piqure: 10mm. Cauterizations: 7—15.
30—BL, Pai Huan Yü.
Piqure: 6—10mm. Cauterizations: FORBIDDEN.
31—BL, Shang Liao.
Piqure: 16—20mm. Cauterizations: 7—15.
32—BL, Tz'u Liao.
Piqure: 16—20mm. Cauterizations: 7—15.
33—BL, Chung Liao.
Piqure: 16—20mm. Cauterizations: 7—15.
34—BL, Hsia Liao.
Piqure: 12—16mm. Cauterizations: 7—15.
35—BL, Hui Yang.
Piqure: 8mm. Cauterizations: 5.

48—BL, Pao Huang.
Piqure: 10—14mm. Cauterizations: 5—10.
49—BL, Chih Pien.
Piqure: 10mm. Cauterizations: 7—15.

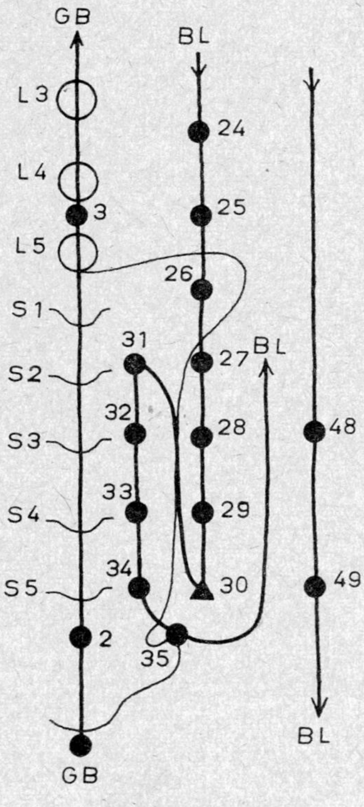

TORSO, sacro-lumbar surface

NECK AND SHOULDER

ANTERIOR SURFACE

9—ST, Jen Yin.
Piqure: FORBIDDEN.
Cauterizations: FORBIDDEN.
10—ST, Shui T'u.
Piqure: 6mm. Cauterizations: 3.
11—ST, Ch'i Shê.
Piqure: 6mm. Cauterizations: 3.
12—ST, Ch'üeh P'en.
Piqure: 6mm. Cauterizations: 3.

21—VC, Hsüan Chi.
Piqure: 6mm. Cauterizations: 5.
22—VC, T'ien T'u.
Piqure: 6mm. Cauterizations: 3—7.
23—VC, Lien Ch'üan.
Piqure: 6mm. Cauterizations: 3—7.

1—LU, Chung Fu.
Piqure: 6—10mm. Cauterizations: 5—10.
2—LU, Yün Men.
Piqure: 6—10mm. Cauterizations: 5—10.

21—GB, Chien Ching.
Piqure: 8—12mm. Cauterizations: 7—15.

Note: For point 27—KI, see THORAX.

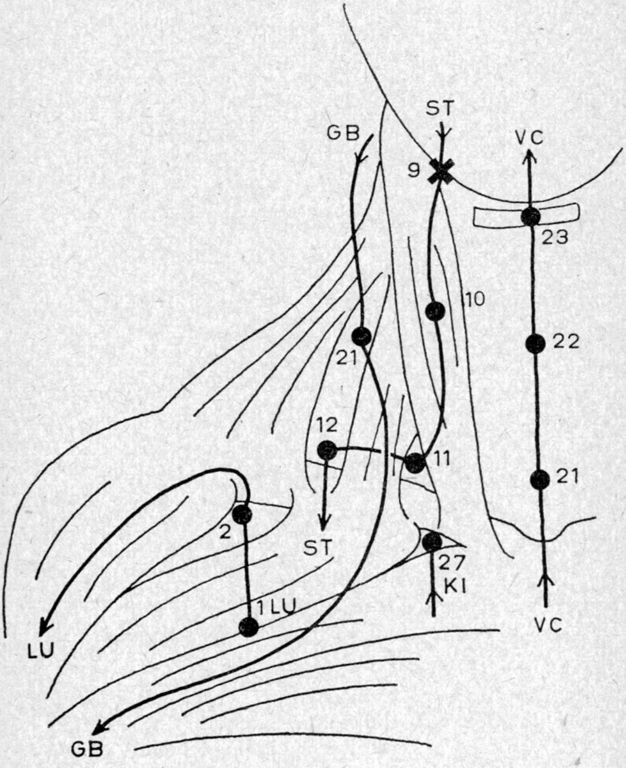

NECK AND SHOULDER, anterior surface

NECK AND SHOULDER

LATERAL SURFACE

15—CO, Chien Yü.
Piqure: 12mm. Cauterizations: 7.

16—CO, Chü Ku.
Piqure: 12mm. Cauterizations: 3—7.

17—CO, T'ien Ting.
Piqure: 6mm. Cauterizations: 3—7.

18—CO, Fu T'u.
Piqure: 8mm. Cauterizations: 3.

16—SI, T'ien Ch'uang.
Piqure: 6mm. Cauterizations: 3.

Note: For point 20—GB, see CRANIUM, the occipup. For points 21—GB, 9—ST, 10—ST, 11—ST, 12—ST, 21—VC, 22—VC and 23—VC, see NECK AND SHOULDER, posterior surface. For point 17—SI, see CRANIUM, the mandible. For point 16—TH, see CRANIUM, the ear.

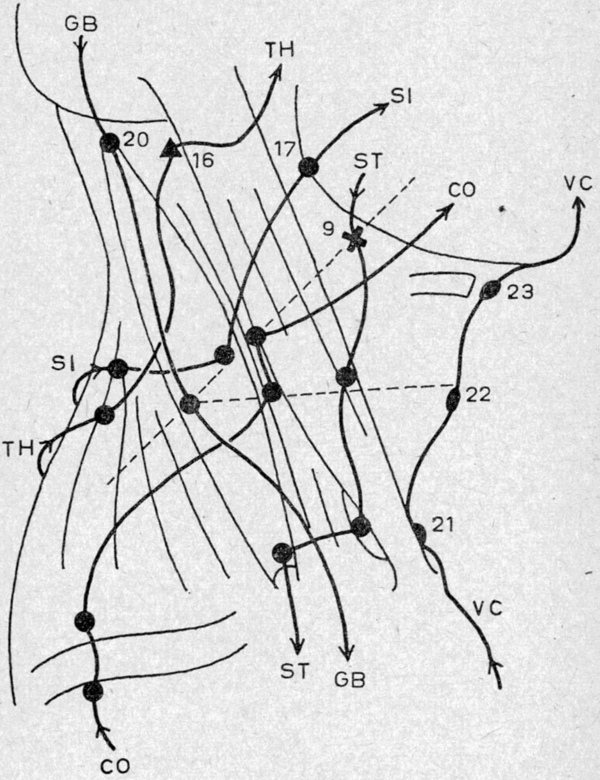

NECK AND SHOULDER, lateral surface

NECK AND SHOULDER

POSTERIOR SURFACE

10—SI, Nao Yü.
Piqure: 10—16mm. Cauterizations: 3—7.
11—SI, T'ien Tsung.
Piqure: 10mm. Cauterizations: 5—7.
12—SI, Ping Fêng.
Piqure: 10mm. Cauterizations: 7.
13—SI, Ch'ü Yüan.
Piqure: 10mm. Cauterizations: 3—7.
14—SI, Chien Wai Yü.
Piqure: 12mm. Cauterizations: 3—10.
15—SI, Chien Chung Yü.
Piqure: 6—12mm. Cauterizations: 5—10.

13—TH, Nao Hui.
Piqure: 10—14mm. Cauterizations: 5—15.
14—TH, Chien Liao.
Piqure: 14mm. Cauterizations: 5—7.
15—TH, T'ien Liao.
Piqure: 6—16mm. Cauterizations: 5—7.

Note: For points 12—VG, 13—VG, 14—VG, 11—BL, 12—BL, 13—BL, 36—BL and 37—BL, see TORSO upper dorsal surface. For points 15—VG, 16—VG, 10—BL and 20—GB, see CRANIUM, the occiput.

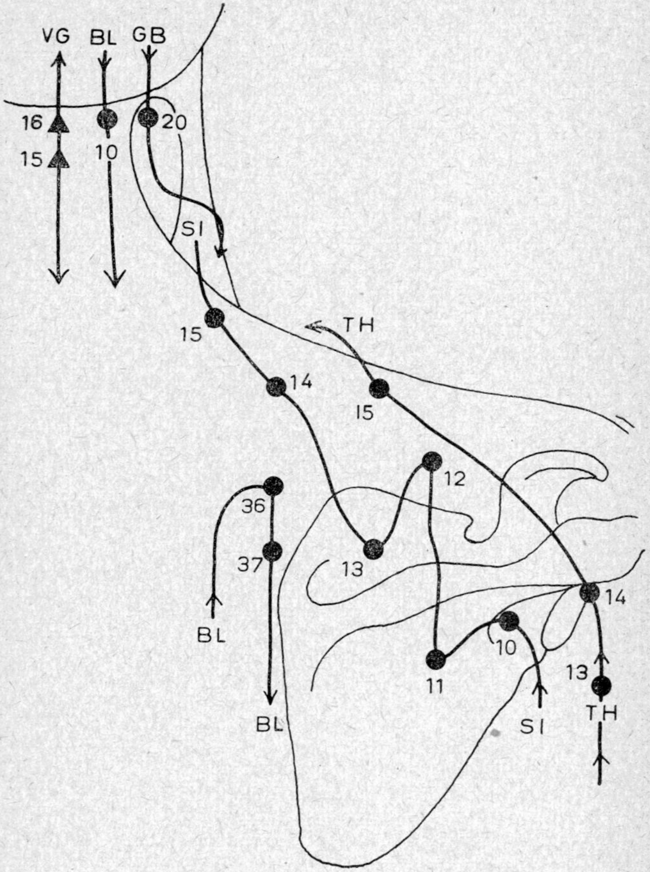

NECK AND SHOULDER, posterior surface

CRANIUM

THE FACE

25—VG, Su Liao.
Piqure: 2mm. Cauterizations: FORBIDDEN.
26—VG, Shui Kou.
Piqure: 4mm. Cauterizations: 3.
27—VG, Yüeh T'uan.
Piqure: 4mm. Cauterizations: 2.

1—BL, Ching Ming.
Piqure: 6mm. Cauterizations: FORBIDDEN.
2—BL, Ts'uan Chu.
Piqure: 4mm. Cauterizations: FORBIDDEN.

19—CO, Ho Liao.
Piqure: 6mm. Cauterizations: FORBIDDEN.
20—CO, Ying Hsiang.
Piqure: 2—6mm. Cauterizations: FORBIDDEN.

1—ST, Ch'eng Chu.
Piqure: FORBIDDEN. Cauterizations: 3.
2—ST, Ssŭ Pai.
Piqure: 6mm. Cauterizations: 3.
3—ST, Chü Liao.
Piqure: 6mm. Cauterizations: 5.
4—ST, Ti T'sang.
Piqure: 6mm. Cauterizations: 5.

24—VC, Ch'eng Chiang.
Piqure: 4—6mm. Cauterizations: 3—7.

1—GB, T'ung Tsŭ Liao.
Piqure: 6mm. Cauterizations: 5.

23—TH, Ssŭ Chu K'ung.
Piqure: 6mm. Cauterizations: FORBIDDEN.

Note: 28—VG, K'en Chiao, is located upon the upper gum and is not shown in the diagram. Its characteristics are: Piqure: 4mm. Cauterizations: 2.

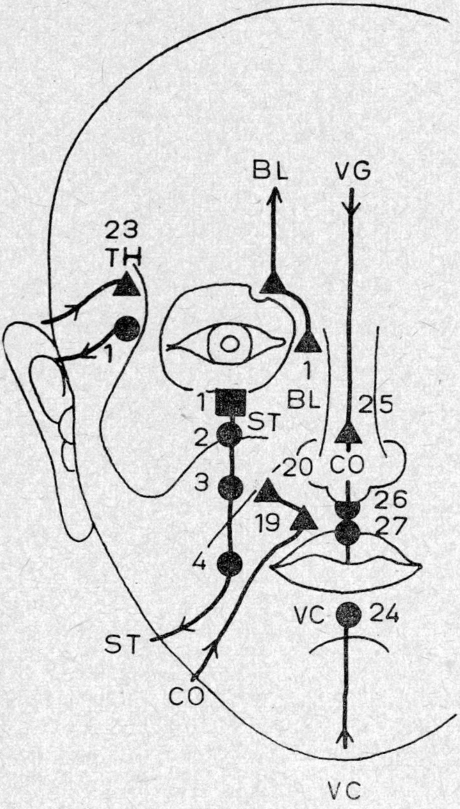

CRANIUM, the face

F

CRANIUM

THE MANDIBLE

5—ST, Ta Ying.
Piqure: 10mm. Cauterizations: 3—5.
6—ST, Chia Chê.
Piqure: 6mm. Cauterizations: 7.
7—ST, Hsia Kuan.
Piqure: 6mm. Cauterizations: FORBIDDEN.

17—SI, T'ien Yung.
Piqure: 6mm. Cauterizations: 3—5.
18—SI, Ch'üan Liao.
Piqure: 6mm. Cauterizations: FORBIDDEN.

Note: For points 2—GB and 19—SI, see CRANIUM, the ear. For points 3—GB, see CRANIUM, the temple.

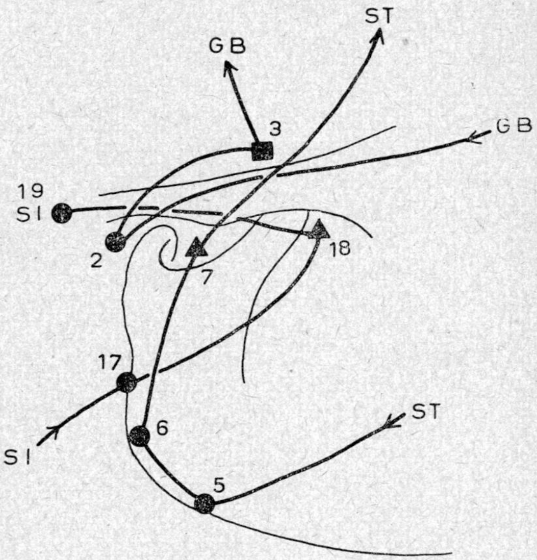

CRANIUM, the mandible

CRANIUM

THE TEMPLE

3—GB, Ko Chu Jen.
Piqure: FORBIDDEN. Cauterizations: 3—5.

4—GB, Han Yen.
Piqure: 4mm. Cauterizations: 3.

5—GB, Hsüan Lu.
Piqure: 6mm. Cauterizations: 3.

6—GB, Hsüan Li.
Piqure: 4mm. Cauterizations: 3.

7—GB, Ch'ü Pin.
Piqure: 6mm. Cauterizations: 3—5.

8—ST, T'ou Wei.
Piqure: 6mm. Cauterizations: FORBIDDEN.

Note: To locate the reference line which extends from point 24—VG to the external auditory meatus (AM), see CRANIUM, co-ordinates and reference points. For point 7—ST, see CRANIUM, the mandible. For point 2—GB, see CRANIUM, the ear.

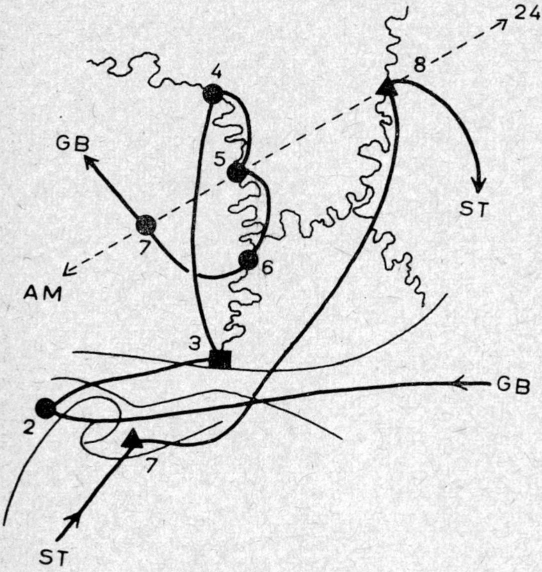

CRANIUM, the temple

CRANIUM

THE EAR

16—TH, T'ien Yu.
Piqure: 6—10mm. Cauterizations: FORBIDDEN.

17—TH, I Fêng.
Piqure: 6mm. Cauterizations: 3—7.

18—TH, Chi Mei.
Piqure: 2mm. Cauterizations: FORBIDDEN.

19—TH, Lu Hsia.
Piqure: FORBIDDEN. Cauterizations: 3—7.

20—TH, Chiao Sun.
Piqure: FORBIDDEN. Cauterizations: 3—7.

21—TH, Erh Men.
Piqure: 6mm. Cauterizations: 6—7.

22—TH, Ho Liao.
Piqure: 6—10mm. Cauterizations: 3—5.

8—GB, Shuai Ku.
Piqure: 6mm. Cauterizations: 3—5.

9—GB, T'ien Ch'ung.
Piqure: 6mm. Cauterizations: 3—5.

10—GB, Fou Pai.
Piqure: 6mm. Cauterizations: 3—5.

11—GB, (T'ou) Ch'ioa Yin.
Piqure: 6mm. Cauterizations: 3—7.

12—GB, Wan Ku.
Piqure: 10mm. Cauterizations: 3—7.

2—GB, T'ing Hui. Piqure: 10mm. Cauterizations: 5.

19—SI, T'ing Kung.
Piqure: 4—6mm. Cauterizations: 3—5.

Note: For point 7—GB, see CRANIUM, the temple.

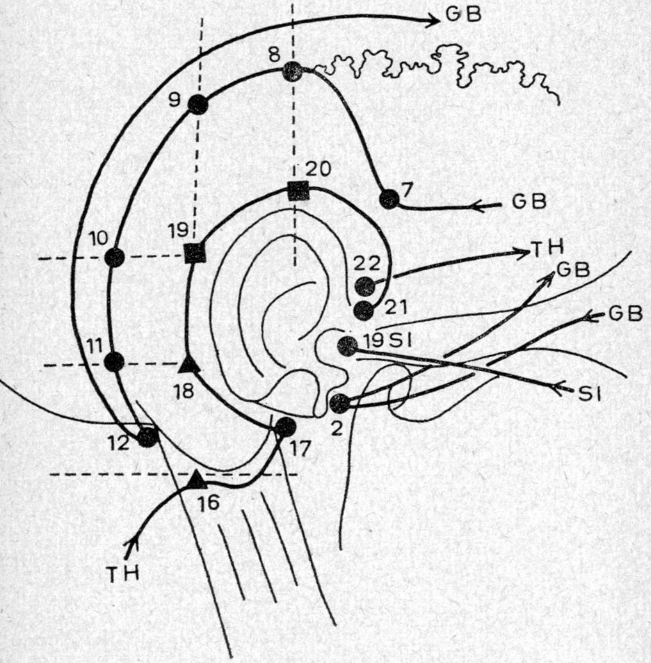

CRANIUM, the ear

CRANIUM

CO-ORDINATES AND REFERENCE POINTS

The meridian of the governing vessel (VG) is on the median line. The local value for the pouce, taken longitudinally, is: 1/18th part of the distance between 14—VG (which is located between the 7th dorsal and 1st thoracic vertebrae) and the glabella (GL).

A line connects the external auditory meatus (AM) with the point 24—VG and separates the region of the forehead from that of the upper cranial region and locates the points 7—GB, 5—GB and 8—ST.

Another line extending from (AM) to the point 20—VG separates the upper cranial region from the occipital region.

15—VG, Ya Men.
Piqure: 6mm. Cauterizations: FORBIDDEN.

16—VG, Fêng Fu.
Piqure: 6mm. Cauterizations: FORBIDDEN.

17—VG, Nao Hu.
Piqure: FORBIDDEN.
Cauterizations: FORBIDDEN.

18—VG, Ch'iang Chien.
Piqure: 4mm. Cauterizations: FORBIDDEN.

19—VG, Hou Ting.
Piqure: 6mm. Cauterizations: 5.

20—VG, Pai Hu.
Piqure: 6mm. Cauterizations: 7.

21—VG, Ch'ien Ting.
Piqure: 4mm. Cauterizations: 3—7.

22—VG, Hsin Hui.
Piqure: 2mm. Cauterizations: 3. Both piqures and cauterizations are FORBIDDEN in the case of children.

23—VG, Shang Hsing.
Piqure: 4mm. Cauterizations: 5.

24—VG, Shen T'ing.
Piqure: FORBIDDEN. Cauterizations: 5.

Note: For point 14—VG see TORSO, upper dorsal region. For points 7—GB, 5—GB and 8—ST see CRANIUM, the temple.

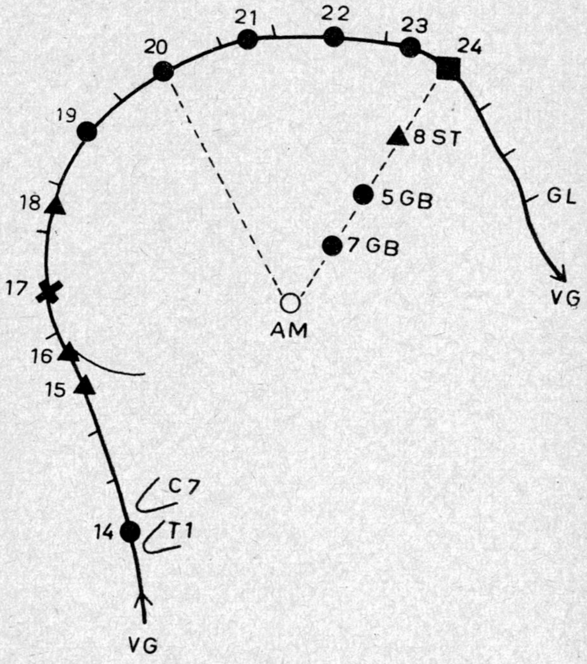

CRANIUM, co-ordinates and reference points

CRANIUM

THE FOREHEAD

3—BL, Mei Chung.
Piqure: 6mm. Cauterizations: 3.
4—BL, Ch'ü Tzŭ.
Piqure: 4mm. Cauterizations: 3—5.

13—GB, Pen Shen.
Piqure: 6mm. Cauterizations: 7.
14—GB, Yang Pai.
Piqure: 5mm. Cauterizations: 3.
15—GB, (T'ou) Lin Ch'i.
Piqure: 6mm. Cauterizations: FORBIDDEN.

Note: For point 8—ST, see CRANIUM, the temple. For points 1—BL and 2—BL, see CRANIUM, the face. For point 24—VG, see CRANIUM, co-ordinates and reference points.

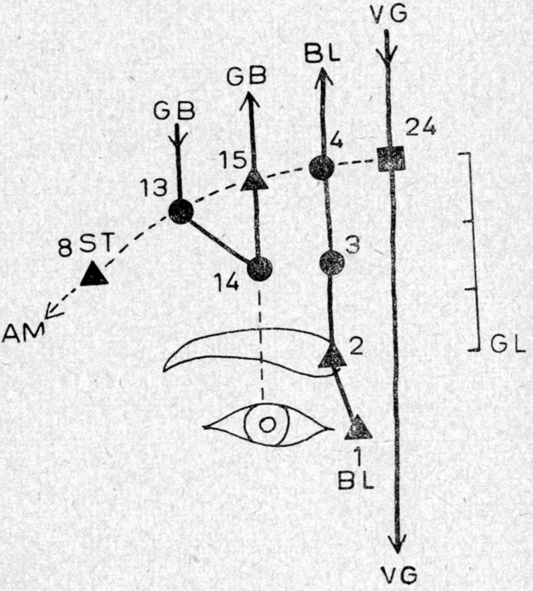

CRANIUM, the forehead

CRANIUM

THE SKULL-CAP

5—BL, Wu Ch'u.
Piqure: 6mm. Cauterizations: FORBIDDEN.
6—BL, Ch'en Kuang.
Piqure: 6mm. Cauterizations: FORBIDDEN.
7—BL, T'ung T'ien.
Piqure: 6mm. Cauterizations: 3—5.

16—GB, Mu Chuang.
Piqure: 6mm. Cauterizations: 5.
17—GB, Cheng Ying.
Piqure: 6mm. Cauterizations: 5.

Note: For points 20—VG, 21—VG, 22—VG, 23—VG and 24—VG, see CRANIUM, co-ordinates and reference points. For points 4—BL, 13—GB and 15—GB, see CRANIUM, the forehead.

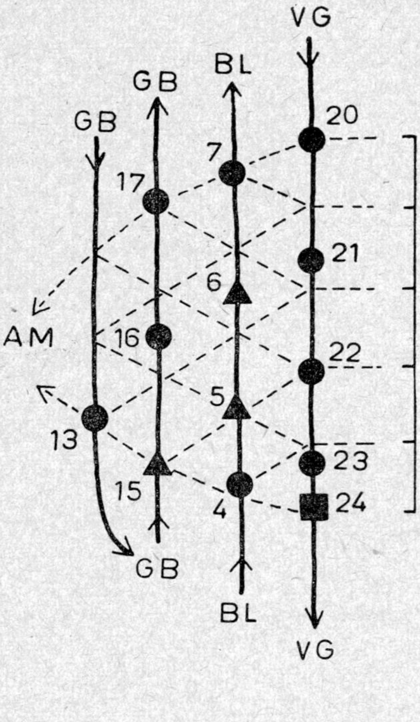

CRANIUM, the skull-cap

CRANIUM

THE OCCIPUT

8—BL, Lê Ch'üeh.
Piqure: 6mm. Cauterizations: 3—5.

9—BL, Yü Chen.
Piqure: 6mm. Cauterizations: 3—5.

10—BL, T'ien Chu.
Piqure: 12mm. Cauterizations: 7—10.

18—GB, Ch'eng Ling.
Piqure: FORBIDDEN. Cauterizations: 5.

19—GB, Nao K'ung.
Piqure: 6mm. Cauterizations: 5.

20—GB, Fêng Ch'ih.
Piqure: 12mm. Cauterizations: 7—10.

Note: For points 15—VG, 16—VG, 17—VG, 18—VG, 19—VG and 20—VG, see CRANIUM, co-ordinates and reference points. For points 7—BL and 17—GB, see CRANIUM, the skull-cap.

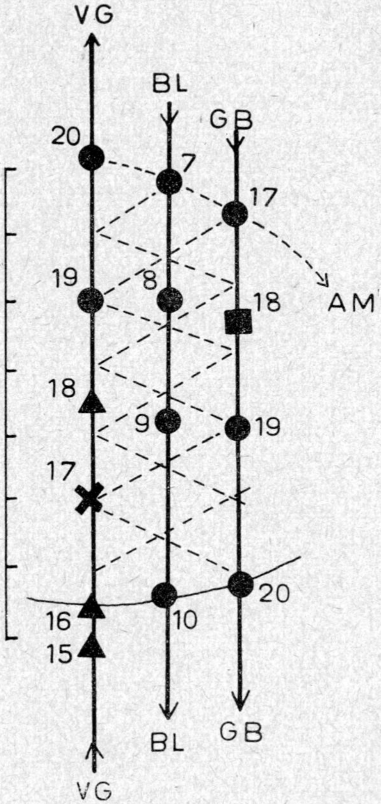

VG
BL
GB
20
7
17
19
8
18
AM
18
9
19
17
20
16
10
15
BL
GB
VG

PART III

BIOENERGY

The relationship between the Yin and the Yang

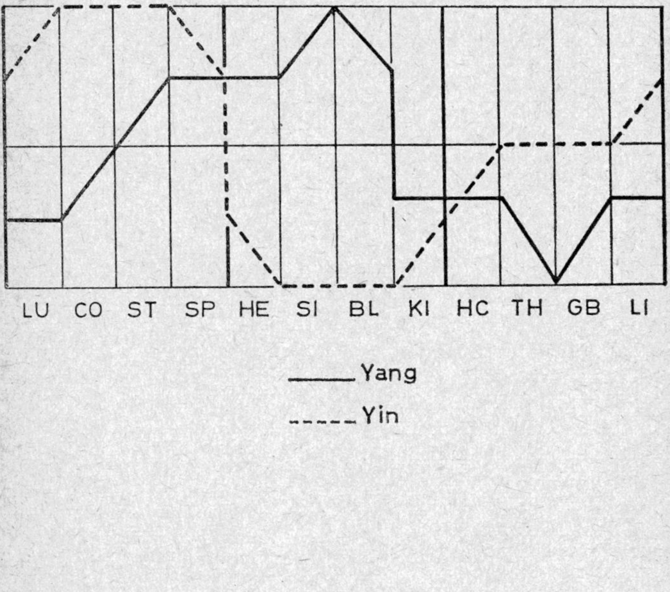

Hsueh Chi, the relationship between the blood and the energy

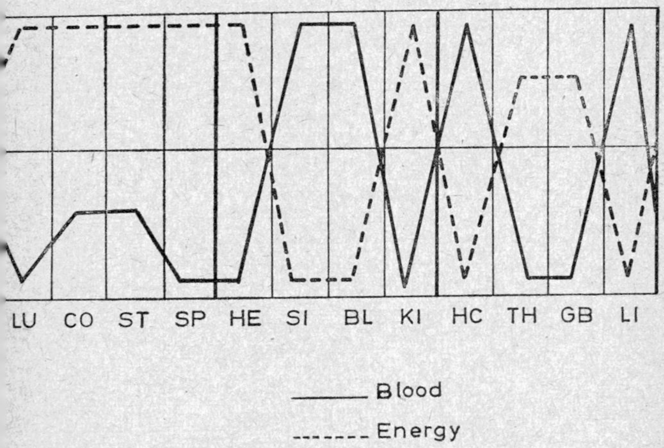

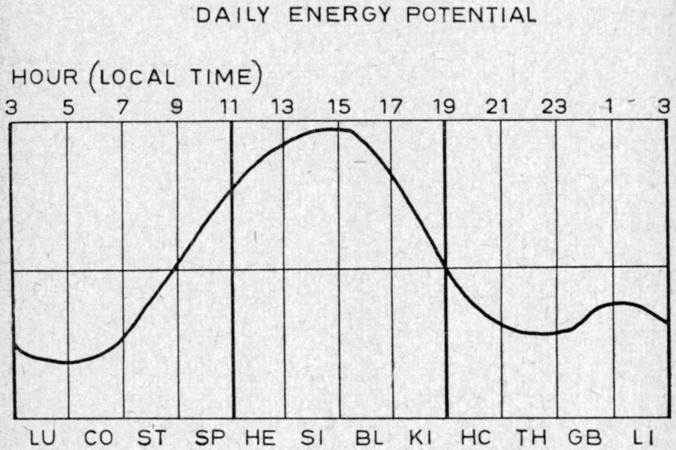

The daily energy potential

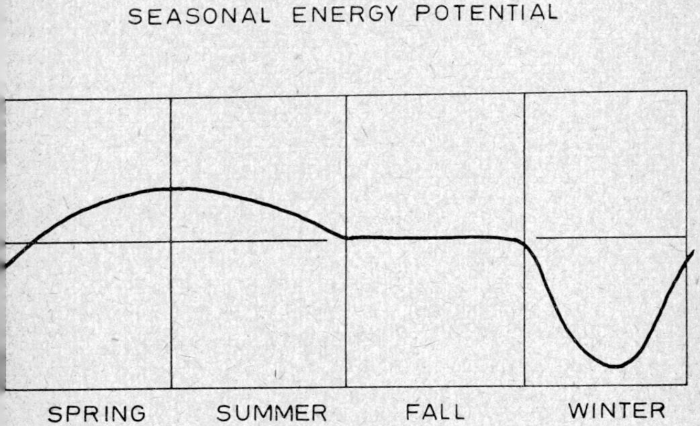

The seasonal energy potential

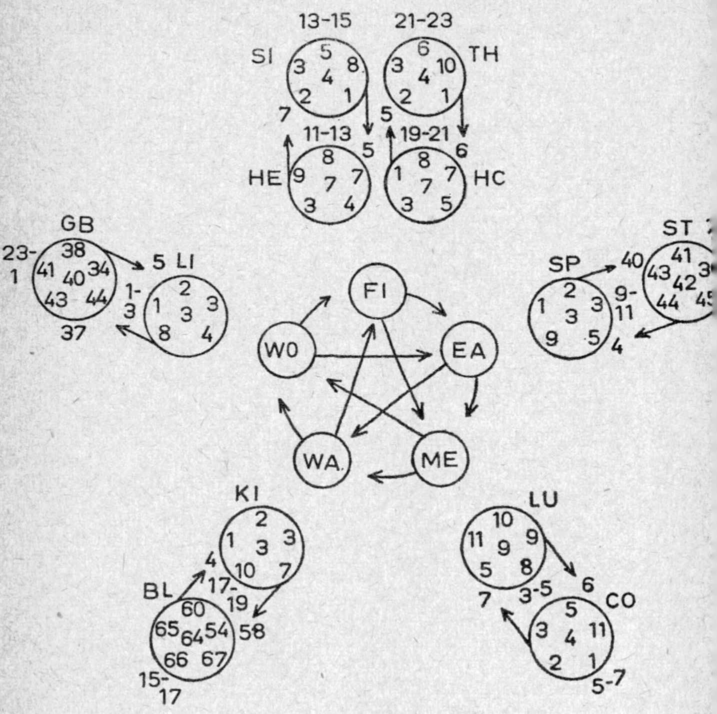

5 Elements. Law of Liu Chu.

Lê Points. Yüen Points. Horary Points.

Diagrams illustrating:

The Five Elements
The Law of Liu Chu
The Lê points
The Yüen points
The Horary points

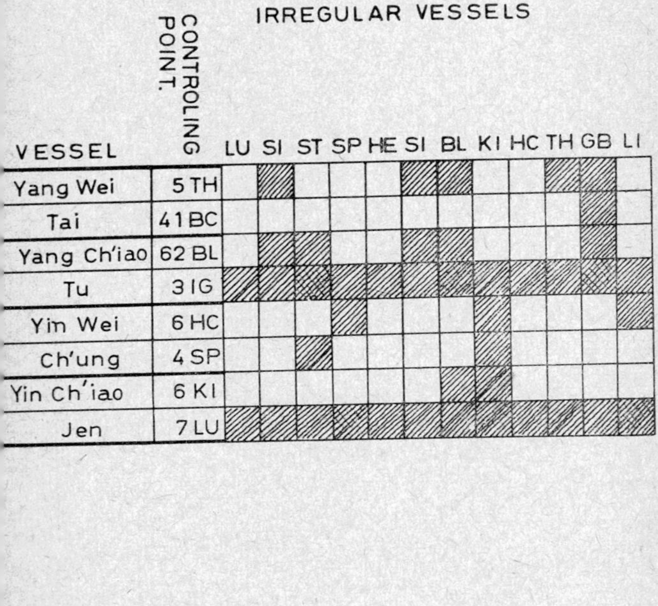

The irregular vessels (Mei)

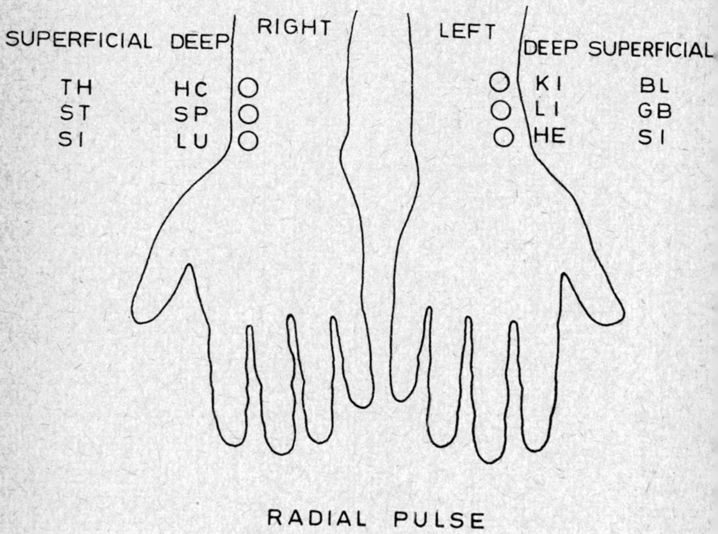

The radial pulse

PART IV

Syntheses of Symptomatic Treatment

Note: This section does not constitute a complete formulary of Acupuncture. The treatments which are outlined here are set forth fully by Dr. Lavier and Dr. Chancellor in their texts **Chinese Acupuncture.**

Rules governing the use of points:

1. Yi Pan Yün Yong Fa.
   Pique local points and distant points.

2. Ten Hsüeh Tu Yong Fa.
   Pique one point only.

3. Shuang Hsüeh Ping Yong Fa.
   Pique two symmetrical points.

4. Sseŭ Chih Hsiang Fa.
   Pique one point on each of the four members.

5. Lien Sou Ping Chen Fa.
   Pique a chain of points upon the same member.

6. Nei Wai Hu Ying Fa.
   Pique points upon the same member, but on opposite surfaces.

7. Luan Huan Chiao T'i Fa.
   Pique to encircle an affected area.

8. Piao Li Hsian P'ei Fa.
   Pique a distal point for an affliction at an opposite extremity.

9. Piao Li Hsian P'ei Fa.
   Pique points in direct rapport with the organ.

10. Tui Cheng Ch'ü Hsüeh Fa.
    Pique the points indicated in the formulary.

Precautions to Be Observed When Treating a Patient:

Always have the patient lie down for treatment.

Check the cardiac and respiratory rhythms; be sure that they are within the normal ratio of 1 : 5.

Never Make a Piqure:

Immediately after a meal.
After any strenuous physical or mental effort.
During a period of anger, of drunkeness, of mortification, or at any time during great excitement.
After coition.
During menstruation.
During pregnancy.
Upon an emaciated patient.
Upon the cranial-suture points of children.
Upon a swelling or an abscess. (See rule 7).
When the moon is full; during high tide if at the seaside.
During a thunderstorm, during a very high wind, or during a hot, sultry day.

Pay Attention to the Points which are Forbidden or Restricted

This precaution applies equally to piqures or cauterizations.

Never Apply a Cauterization when the Pulse is Lower than 30 or Higher than 80.

Avoid cauterizing the Epigastrium area too often.

GENERAL PRINCIPLES OF MAKING A PIQURE:

	Pou Stimulates	Hsieh Calms
Pique:	slowly	rapidly
Leave needle in place for a:	short time	long time
Withdraw:	rapidly	slowly
After treatment:	massage the piqure	do not massage the piqure

If the meridian contains more blood than energy, allow it to bleed.

If the meridian contains more energy than blood, do not allow it to bleed. (See the relationship of Hsueh-Chi, page 87.)

ORGANS, TISSUES AND THE FIVE ELEMENTS

	Wood	Fire	Earth	Metal	Water
Tsang:	LI	HE+HC	SP	LU	KI
Fou (coupled):	GB	SI+TH	ST	CO	BL
Organ:	Eye	Tongue	Mouth	Nose	Ear
Tissue:	Muscle	Vessels	Conjunctivia	Skin	Bones

GENERAL STIMULATION OF THE BODY

Rule 2:

36—ST, to stimulate the energy in general.
16—BL, to stimulate the organs.
38—BL, for chronic disease.
46—BL, for chronic mental affections.
12—BL, as a prophylactic after exposure to cold.

Rule 10:

14—GB, 4—CO, 11—CO.
11—CO, 34—GB.
6—11, 6—SP after a depressing disease.

SKIN AND MUSCLES

Skin:

Rule 7: Locally.
Rule 10: 11—CO, 6—SP.
For the Five Elements: 13—BL.

Muscles:

For the Five Elements: 18—BL.
Rule 10: Shoulder and arms: 11—CO, 15—CO.
Buttocks and leg: 30—GB, 34—GB.

Infiltration:

Rule 2: 9—VC.

H

RHEUMATISM

The first attack.

Apply Rule 4. Pique 11—CO and 54—BL.
If on the lower members, add 39—ST.
If on the upper members, add 8—SI.

Chronic rheumatism.

Rule 7. ...

For the shoulder and scapular area: 15—CO, 12—SI, 11—CO, 10—CO and 11—BL.

For the lumbar area: 47—BL and 25—BL. Add 54—BL to accord with rules 1 and 2.

For the back: 13—VG and 9—VG. Add 54—BL to accord with rules 1 and 2.

For the buttocks: 30—GB.

For the thigh: 31—GB.

For the knee: 34—GB and 53—BL.

For the leg: 57—BL and 6—SP.

For the arms: 14—CO.

For the elbow: 11—CO and 5—LU.

For the forearm: 10—CO.

For the neck: 20—VG and 16—VG. Add 7—LU to accord with rules 1 and 2.

For the face: 6—ST, 4—ST and 2—BL. Add 4—CO to accord with rules 1 and 2.

Do not forget the special technique for this malady: Hsieh for the duration of the attack. Pou for the heat. If there is tumefaction, it is advisable to apply Rule 7.

RESPIRATORY SYSTEM

Rule 2:

For the prevention of the effects of chilling: 12—BL.
For asthma: 22—VC.
For chronic maladies and pulmonary afflictions: 38—BL.

Point of command:
For the lungs: 13—BL.

Special points for the trachea and bronchii:
22—VC, 12—BL, 13—BL and 40—ST.

Rule 10:
General formula for the respiratory system: 10—LU and 3—KI.
For bronchitis, cough and dyspnea: 4—CO, 11—LU and 1—CO.
For the trachea and throat: 11—CO and 15—CO.
For pleurisy: 14—VG and 6—HC.

GENITO-URINARY SYSTEM

Rule 2:

Genito-urinary points: 5—VC and 6—VC.

The genital points are: 6—SP, the points of the sacral foramena and 47—BL.

Local genital points are: 7—VC, 29—ST and 30—ST with 3—VC and 4—VC.

Rule 10:

General formula for the genito-urinary system: 6—VC and 25—ST.

General formula for the uterus and ovaries: 11—CO and 6—SP.

NERVOUS SYSTEM

Rule 2:

Psychopathies: 20—VG or 7—HE.
Nervous insomnia: 45—ST.
Headaches: 7—LU.
Dorsal-lumbar pains: 54—BL.
Medullary and cerebral afflictions: 12—VG.

Rule 10:

General formula to calm the nervous system: 4—CO, 3—LI.

In the case of a mental derangement, add: 40—ST and 34—GB.

If the mental derangement is very serious (such as epilepsy or convulsions), add: 2—VG and 7—HE.

Neuralgias and paralysis:

Apply Rules: 1, 5, 6, 7 and 8.

In the case of paralysis, remember to treat the healthy side of the body.

THE MOUTH

Rule 2:

Pique 4—CO.

Buccal mucous membranes:

Rule 10: 11—CO, 4—CO, 26—VG and 8—HC.
Regional points: 10—BL, 20—GB and 14—VG.
Local points: 4—ST, 6—ST and 28—VG.

Tongue:

For the Five Elements: 15—BL.
Rule 2: 7—CO.
Local point: 23—VC.

Teeth:

Rule 2: 44—ST (toothache).
For the Five Elements: 23—BL.
Local points: Located upon the face.

EYE, EAR, NOSE AND THROAT

Eye:

For the Five Elements: 18—BL.
Rule: 10: 11—CO, 4—CO, 1—BL and 23—TH.
Rule 2: 36—ST.

Ear:

For the Five Elements: 23—BL.
Rule 10: 11—CO, 4—CO, 2—GB and 17—TH.
Regional points: 20—GB.

Nose:

For the Five Elements: 13—BL.
Rule 10: 11—CO, 4—CO, 19—CO and 20—CO.
Regional points: 7—BL and 23—VG.
Rhinitis: 10—BL, 2—GB.
Epistaxis: 23—VG and 54—BL.

Throat:

Rule 2: 8—LU (pharynx)
17—CO (throat)
Rule 10: 11—CO, 4—CO, 6—ST and 10—LU.
Larynx: 22—VC and 8—LU.
Tonsils: 17—SI and 17—CO.

DIGESTIVE TRACT

Rule 2:

For all affections of the digestive tract: 36—ST.
Acute gastritis: 21—ST.
Chronic diarrhea: 25—ST.
Constipation: 2—CO.
Vomiting: in children: 19—TH.

Rule 10:

For all gastro-intestinal afflictions: 6—SP and 36—ST.

Hypotonea and sluggishness of the digestive tract: 4—CO and 36—ST.

Maladies of the stomach: 8—HC and 36—ST.

Constipation: 40—ST and 34—GB.

Vomiting and diarrhea: 12—VC and 36—ST; if necessary bleed 3—HC and 54—BL. After the symptoms have disappeared, follow by piqures at 6—HC and 6—SP for general stimulation.

Points of command:

Liver: 18—BL.
Gall Bladder: 19—BL.
Stomach: 21—BL.
Colon: 25—BL.
Small Intestine: 27—BL.

Local or metametric points:

Upper Esophagus: 2—VC.
Lower Esophagus: 12—VC and 17—BL.
Pylorus: 10—VC and 21—BL.
Stomach: 11—VC, 12—VC and 21—BL.
Cardia: 13—VC and 21—BL.
Liver: 12—VC, 14—VC and on the right side: 13—LI, 14—LI, 18—BL and 19—BL.
Pancreas: 12—VC and on the left side: 17—BL, 18—BL and 19—BL.
Gall Bladder: 12—VC, 9—VG and on the right side: 13—LI, and 19—BL.
Intestines: 9—VC, 4—VC, 24—ST and 4—VG.

Note: 6—HC always reinforces, from a distance, the effects of 12—VC.

Special Index of Points

By Dr. PHILIP M. CHANCELLOR

The number of the point and the page on which it is listed.

Stomach (ST).

1	68	24	50
2	68	25	50
3	68	26	52
4	68	27	52
5	70	28	52
6	70	29	52
7	70	30	52
8	72	31	24
9	62	32	24
10	62	33	24
11	62	34	24
12	62	35	24
13	48	36	32
14	48	37	32
15	48	38	32
16	48	39	32
17	48	40	32
18	48	41	32
19	50	42	42
20	50	43	42
21	50	44	42
22	50	45	42
23	50		

Bladder (BL)

1	68
2	68
3	73
4	73
5	80
6	80
7	80
8	82
9	82
10	82
11	56
12	56
13	56
14	56
15	56
16	56
17	56
18	58
19	58
20	58
21	58
22	58
23	58
24	60
25	60
26	60
27	60
28	60
29	60
30	60
31	60
32	60
33	60
34	60
35	60
36	56
37	56
38	56
39	56
40	56
41	56
42	58
43	58
44	58
45	58
46	58
47	58
48	60
49	60
50	26
51	26
52	26
53	26
54	26
55	34
56	34
57	34
58	36
59	36
60	44
61	44
62	44
63	44
64	44
65	44
66	44
67	44

Kidneys (KI).

1	46
2	46
3	46
4	46
5	46
6	46
7	38
8	38
9	38
10	30
11	52
12	52
13	52
14	52
15	52
16	50
17	50
18	50
19	50
20	50
21	50
22	48
23	48
24	48
25	48
26	48
27	48

Heart Constrictor (HC)

1	8
2	8
3	8
4	14
5	14
6	14
7	14
8	20
9	22

Tri-heaters (TH)

1	22
2	22
3	22
4	16
5	16
6	16
7	16
8	16
9	16
10	10
11	10
12	10
13	66
14	66
15	66
16	74
17	74
18	74
19	74
20	74
21	74
22	74
23	68

Small Intestine (SI).

1	22
2	22
3	22
4	22
5	16
6	16
7	16
8	16
9	10
10	66
11	66
12	66
13	66
14	66
15	66
16	64
17	70
18	70
19	74

Gallbladder (GB).

1	68
2	74
3	72
4	72
5	72
6	72
7	72
8	74
9	74
10	74
11	74
12	74
13	78
14	78
15	78
16	80
17	80
18	82
19	82
20	82
21	62
22	54
23	54
24	50
25	54
26	54
27	54
28	54
29	54
30	28
31	28
32	28
33	28
34	36
35	36
36	36
37	36
38	36
39	36
40	44
41	42
42	42
43	42
44	42

Liver (LI).

1	42
2	42
3	42
4	42
5	38
6	38
7	38
8	30
9	30
10	24
11	52
12	52
13	54
14	50

Vessel of conception (VC).

1	52
2	52
3	52
4	52
5	52
6	52
7	52
8	50
9	50
10	50
11	50
12	50
13	50
14	50
15	50
16	48
17	48
18	48
19	48
20	48
21	62
22	62
23	62
24	68

Governing vessel
(VG).

1	60
2	60
3	60
4	58
5	58
6	58
7	58
8	58
9	56
10	56
11	56
12	56
13	56
14	56
15	76
16	76
17	76
18	76
19	76
20	76
21	76
22	76
23	76
24	76
25	68
26	68
27	68
28	68

Printed by
The Albion Press,
223/225 Central Road,
Morden, Surrey.